SUPPORTING FAT BIRTH

by the same author

Supporting Queer Birth
A Book for Birth Professionals and Parents
AJ Silver
ISBN 978 1 83997 045 0
eISBN 978 1 83997 046 7

of related interest

Stretched to the Limits
Supporting Women with Hypermobile Ehlers-Danlos Syndrome
(hEDS) Through Pregnancy, Labour, and Postnatally
Rachel Fitz-Desorgher
ISBN 978 1 83997 249 2
eISBN 978 1 83997 250 8

Supporting Autistic People Through Pregnancy and Childbirth
Hayley Morgan, Emma Durman and Karen Henry
ISBN 978 1 83997 105 1
eISBN 978 1 83997 106 8

Supporting Survivors of Sexual Abuse Through Pregnancy and Childbirth
A Guide for Midwives, Doulas and Other Healthcare Professionals
Kicki Hansard
Forewords by Penny Simkin and Phyllis Klaus
ISBN 978 1 84819 424 3
eISBN 978 0 85701 377 4

Supporting Fat Birth

Supporting Body Positive Birth

AJ Silver

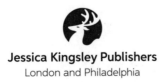

Jessica Kingsley Publishers
London and Philadelphia

First published in Great Britain in 2024 by Jessica Kingsley Publishers
An imprint of John Murray Press

1

INSERT any disclaimers

A CIP catalogue record for this title is available from the British Library and the
Library of Congress

ISBN 978 1 83997 633 9
eISBN 978 1 83997 634 6

Printed and bound in Great Britain by TJ Books Ltd

Jessica Kingsley Publishers' policy is to use papers that are natural, renewable
and recyclable products and made from wood grown in sustainable forests.
The logging and manufacturing processes are expected to conform to the
environmental regulations of the country of origin.

Jessica Kingsley Publishers
Carmelite House
50 Victoria Embankment
London EC4Y 0DZ

www.jkp.com

John Murray Press
Part of Hodder & Stoughton Ltd
An Hachette Company

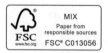

MIX
Paper from
responsible sources
FSC® C013056

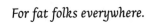

For fat folks everywhere.

Contents

	Preface	9
Ch 1:	Intro	11
Ch 2:	Fat, Black and Pregnant	34
Ch 3:	Conception	49
Ch 4:	Fat, Black, Queer and considering conceiving	66
Ch 5:	Fat Birth	79
Ch 6:	Fat and Multipara	88
Ch 7:	Pregnancy and Birth Choices	106
Ch 8:	Big Birthas	110
Ch 9:	Gestational Diabetes	134
Ch 10:	Water Birth	145
Ch 11:	Home Birth	150
Ch 12:	Induction of Labour	160
Ch 13:	Perinatal and Fat	177
Ch 14:	Fat Parenting	194
Ch 15:	Rebuttals, Objections and Advocacy	206
	Afterword	216
	Index	217

Preface

Before we get right in about it, let me tell you first about the language I use in this book and its intended audience. Throughout I use a variety of words to refer to pregnant women and pregnant people. I use language that is, as far as possible, inclusive of all who become pregnant and who birth their babies. This may be mothers and women, trans men, non-binary people assigned female at birth (like me!), intersex folks or anyone else who is not a cisgender (someone who does identify with the sex they were assigned at birth) woman. I covered the reasons why this is important in my first book, *Supporting Queer Birth*, and won't spend these first few chapters walking over my own footsteps. However, gender inclusive language is a seemingly increasingly controversial subject. I know, I know – including all who experience parenthood and birth isn't controversial in the slightest. But some do see the inclusion of trans men, non-binary folk assigned female at birth and the wider LGBTQ+ community as not just an inconvenient necessity, but also as an affront, that our inclusion works in resistance to the goal: the goal being that all service users be given access to individualized and humanizing care in maternity and perinatal services.

I am an advocate for additive language: using a mixture of language to reflect the mixture of service users. No two women or people experience the same conception, pregnancy, birth or perinatal period; no two pregnant women or other pregnant people will want or need the same treatment, support and guidance as any other. You will hear stories and experiences from various service users as well as healthcare professionals and birth workers. Some of them are women and mothers; some are transgender and non-binary. We will also hear from non-gestational parents, mothers and fathers. As most people will agree, having a solid supporting team or birthing partner can improve experiences. These may be non-gestational parents and/ or birth professionals such as doulas. Excluding the experience of non-gestational parents would mean that we were losing elements of the story. And we will also hear from fat professionals who may or may not be parents themselves.

My role is to serve as your doula on this journey. You may be a fat or a straight-sized birth worker wondering how anti-fat bias is affecting your ability to give good care or how it affects the experience of fat service users. Or you may be a fat person considering starting or expanding your family and wondering how to equip yourself with as much information as possible.

However you arrived here, welcome.

CHAPTER 1

Intro

This clearly isn't a textbook, but we *will* talk about some stats and statistics. However, the most important part is asking yourself the hard questions. I am a huge believer in asking 'Who told you that?' In all kinds of external and internal conversations and investigations, checking my sourcing has proved invaluable.

Who told me that it was only my weight contributing to my pain? Sometimes it was healthcare professionals directly, but more often indirectly. It may have come from being continually told that I was a fat ticking time bomb, and although 'for now', they'd say, my blood pressure, HbA1c (blood sugar level) results or whatever else I am being tested for has come back within range, at some point my fat will implode into my body and cause pain, suffering and possibly even death.

From what clothes I can wear to which seats are built with folks like me in mind, to where I can give birth, what services I can and can't be referred to based on my body mass index (BMI), and on and on it goes.

We need to begin talking about why *fat* birth matters. If we settle for 'plus size', we are placing the default, the expected, the normal at 'straight sized'.

Straight sized: folks who fall into the societal expectation of average, default-sized bodies.

'Plus size', by its very nature, means more than expected, more than normal. If we remove the centralization of straight-sized bodies as normal, then plus size folks aren't normal *plus* – we are fat. Plus size may be more palatable, more PG-13, less invasive in a world that centres straight-sized bodies and vilifies those in larger bodies. But, in a fat-neutral or fat-positive world, 'fat' isn't a bad word. Fat isn't an insult. Fat isn't negative. Fat isn't less than. Fat isn't worse. *Fat is healthy, fat is sexy, fat is neutrality, fat is fabulous.*

As with many instances of reclamation of language (see 'slut', 'queer' etc.),[1] 'fat' can and often does immediately spark discomfort. Fat has been used as an insult in western culture for aeons – from 'Your mama is so fat' to 'fat bitch', those of us who exist in larger-than-expected or -defaulted bodies have heard it all. Reclamation of language is a powershift. No longer content to be beaten with these weaponized words, we'll grab that stick you beat us with, and now that we are holding it, empowered by it, fucking thriving with it, it can no longer be wielded as before.

Even if overnight anti-fat bias disappeared from our conscious and unconscious selves, we would still live in a world that doesn't expect fat folks to be there. This may look like *body-positive* brands that make their *redefine beauty* t-shirts up to a size 20 (if you're lucky, most often a size 18), often having them modelled by straight-sized models and editing the pictures, or even providing straight-sized models with padding, ahem, I mean fat suits, to acquire the (sometimes) acceptable or desirable parts of fat bodies – thick thighs, big boobs – but leaving out the undesirable – arm fat, double chins, back rolls. It may look like medical providers not having dignity wear or blood pressure cuffs in sizes for all their clients. So, plus size serves to reframe fat bodies as normal bodies *plus* extra, rather than standalone, accepted, gloriously fat bodies.

When you read or hear the word 'fat' as a descriptor, what happens internally for you?

Common rebuttals I experience at almost every instance of naming myself as 'fat' include, but are not limited to: 'You aren't fat, you are

---

1   www.dictionary.com/e/reclaiming-controversial-terms

beautiful!' Never said I wasn't beautiful – I said I was fat. The two aren't diametric poles that can never touch; they do, often.

'Don't be so hard on yourself!' Again, implying fat is negative or undesirable. Perhaps reinvest that toxic kindness into asking venues with tiny chairs why they don't want fat folks in their space.

'You can lose weight, though! They will *always* be ugly, no matter how skinny...' Holy internalized fatphobia, Batman! First, body size isn't a prerequisite for beauty or desirability. If you believe that losing, or indeed gaining, weight would make someone more acceptable, ask yourself: 'Who told me that? Who benefits from diet culture? Who suffers?' Second, who is 'they'? Straight-sized folk? Why are they ugly? Who told you this? Fat liberation only exists in a sphere of decentralization of the 'perfect body', which changes across time, geography, cultures and society.

'As long as you are happy and healthy, that's all that matters...' I can't quite muster a big enough eye roll for this one. Body size and health are not strictly paired factors. If your acceptance or even neutrality of fat folks hinges on our being healthy, you may need to explore your ableism further. The thinly veiled defence of concern for fat people's health falls apart rather quickly when you remove the base coding of size = health.

Sometimes naming or describing myself as 'fat' may even elicit the glorifying obesity remarks. Before we pull this apart with the vigour of a tear-to-share garlic bread, let's pause for a quick explanation of levels of fatness. Not everyone uses these categories or labels, but acknowledging that the levels of restrictions or fatphobia that we experience are based on a spectrum of acceptability is important. The further you are from societal acceptable sizing, the greater you may experience the restrictions and effects of fatphobia:

- Straight-sized: Someone who exists unencumbered by society's framing of 'normal' or 'average' body sizes. This may look like someone who can purchase clothes in high street stores largely unaffected by fatphobia, someone whose weight is not used as a catch-all for blame in medical settings, and who can largely exist without consideration of their size restricting their choices or options.

- Small fat/skinny fat: This person may start to struggle in some stores to find clothing in a UK 18+ size, although brands differ. They may experience medical or size discrimination in some instances, but can largely participate in life with few restrictions based on their size.
- Middle fat/mid fat: They are typically restricted in their choice of brands, stores and styles. Think stripes babe, and plaid, lots of plaid. (When even the bisexuals are saying it's too much plaid, you know it really is too much plaid.) They may have trouble fitting in seats or spaces that are designed for the expected, default body size. They may find more frequent investigations into their health and wellbeing scapegoat their size as the cause.
- Large fat/mega fat: This person may be at the uppermost of plus size clothing brands. They are heavily restricted in their choices and in navigating spaces. The main focus of their healthcare is on their weight and diet. They are often restricted in accessibility based on their size.
- Super-fat/infinity fat: Super-fat folk may experience significant barriers to access healthcare, fashion and wider access needs such as seating.

Of course, not all folks existing in larger bodies use the same language to describe themselves. If your joy resides in terminology such as plus size, fluffy, thicc, chunky, chubby, portly, dumpy, big, rotund, heavy, stout, plump, burly, paunchy, corpulent or husky, then follow your joy.

While exploring these *fat-agories* and variation in treatment and experiences based on body size, consider also intersectionality. Anti-Blackness, colourism, anti-LGBTQ+, Islamophobia, antisemitism, ageism, ableism and classism all intersect with how people are treated as they exist throughout the world. Claiming that fatphobia doesn't impact the lives of folks who can walk into high street retailers and grab their size with ease doesn't erase the other intersections of their identities. (Try and find an off-the-peg suit for fat trans masculine people. No, go ahead, I'll wait.) It also doesn't serve to dismantle the systems of oppression for fat folk.

Fatphobia doesn't only impact women and people assigned female at birth.

People assigned female at birth: folks who were assigned female at birth, but who do not identify with their assigned-at-birth gender. Trans men and non-binary folks, for example.

While usually cisgender men's fashion exists in the realm of *big and tall* rather than 'plus size' (your misogyny is showing, babe), men are still impacted by anti-fatness and fatphobia.

Applying the above, we can see how *body positivity* reserved almost exclusively for small, fat, cisgender, white, middle-class women may be the extent of radical fat acceptance for some brands, people and societies. Have a look on Etsy for body-positive slogan clothing, and see how many go above size 24. Again, I will wait.

Of course, the focus on availability of fashion isn't the most urgent of disparities faced by fat folks across the globe. However, it is a tangible and relatable experience for folks in everyday life.

BMI is bullshit

Take your weight in kilograms, divide by your height in metres squared, and out pops a number.

If that is between 18.5 and 25, you are considered to have a healthy BMI (body mass index); 25–30: you are overweight. And on it goes.

On one visual I found on Diabetes UK (that I found to be particularly tooth itch-inducing), a vertical axis shows height in feet and inches with the horizontal axis showing weight in pounds and kilograms, increasing left to right. The diagonal lines that divide 'Underweight', 'Normal', 'Overweight', 'Obese' and 'Morbidly obese' are coloured for our convenience. White and neutral for 'Underweight'. Green for 'Go ahead, live your life' 'Normal'. Yellow, 'Get ready to stop' 'Overweight'. Orange for 'Holy shit it's getting to concerning' 'Obese'. And, of course, red for 'Fucking stop eating now' 'Morbidly obese'. And if that wasn't helpful enough, we also have illustrated stick figures running from the slightly hall of mirrors underweights to an overweight and then morbidly obese 'stick' figure circa Violet Beauregarde: 'You are turning violet, Violet!' Roll me away to Mr Wonka's deflator circular.

Quetelet created the equation of body weight divided by height squared, this was known as the Quetelet index until it was renamed as BMI in 1972. Quetelet formed the basis of his calculations and categories using exclusively White, cisgender, non-disabled, male western Europeans, although to be clear, he did say it shouldn't be used as a measure of individual health. We must also remember Quetelet's work and belief in eugenics.[2]

But here we are, in 2023, using BMI on all folks, regardless of sex or race, as a checklist of requirements to get treatment – lifesaving treatment in some cases. From access to conception services like IVF to perceived choice of place of birth, the list goes on.

Some maternity and perinatal trusts assert the 30+ BMI = high-risk 'cut-off', while in another hospital down the road it's 35+ BMI = high-risk pregnancy, even though research in 2010[3] concluded that there was 'insufficient evidence, at present, to deny women fertility treatment on grounds of BMI'. You'll be forgiven, as a fat person moving through perinatal services, for thinking there were huge oceans of proof that fat = dangerous.

For folks who have lived without weight stigma, it can be difficult to fathom just how much of an impact it has on your daily life.

Around the time my father died in April 2020, I started to experience back pain, a random, gnawing intermittent pain. I assumed that between the lockdown restrictions and my grief I had stopped moving and I was seizing up. Speaking to my spouse, he mused if getting back to my yoga would be beneficial with the lack of movement in lockdown, and to see when the chiropractor was reopening and could squeeze me in. This might be the end of the train of thought for some,

---

2   https://academic.oup.com/ndt/article/23/1/47/1923176?login=false
3   https://academic.oup.com/humrep/article/25/4/815/700269, p.818.

but, as a fat person who has lived for 32 years being told that their fat is the cause of most, if not all, their health conditions, it wasn't.

Despite my wonderful chiropractor, sports massage therapist, talking therapy and moving for a minimum of 14,000 steps a day (this was no mean feat when we were only allowed out once a day for an hour, in the strictest of lockdown measures), my pain wasn't going away; in fact, it was getting worse.

Given my previous experiences of healthcare professionals blaming my complaints on my fat, it took me 18 months to finally get to the point that even at the risk of being diagnosed as 'fat' again, I had to go to my doctor. My back pain had migrated to my stomach, and, apologies if you are eating, but I hadn't had a solid movement in months. Eating grilled chicken breast and boiled rice only to be relieved of any stomach contents within minutes of completing a meal, I can wholeheartedly attest, fucks with your mind. Continually hungry, scared to eat in case you spend the following hours making best friends with your loo, isn't fun. Finding a GP who didn't immediately ask my weight before any other questions was the small dream I held on to. I was not ready for Dr Z. He was my angel.

He listened to me, he palpated me, he asked after my emotional wellbeing, and rather than assume that I lived on fast food, he asked if these pain 'attacks' synced up with my eating schedule or if had noticed any sync up with certain foods. He even placed his hand on my arm as I began to sob with relief and gratitude that he had not already dispatched me from the surgery clutching a WeightWatchers voucher. He reassured me that I need not fear being diagnosed as fat by him, and that not only was that the refuge of lazy healthcare professionals, but it was also not, in his view, the cause of my health problems.

One ridiculously fast referral to ultrasound later, there they were... an actual reason my body was hurting. A reason other than the thought I had that my 20-stone body was crushing my spine because I was so large: gallstones.

For 18 months I had been in pain. Such pain that I had taken myself to Accident & Emergency, imagined cutting the pain out of my useless body, and dreaded waking up in the mornings, the twisting and turning in bed waking both my spouse and the dog. She would (the dog that is) lift her head from the bed, sniff, nudge and finally lick my face as if to say 'I love you, but I can't sleep like this' before alighting the bed while ensuring her huff of displeasure was vocalized. Waking to take my children to school or go to work (mostly both), I was completely discombobulated from lack of sleep, lack of sound and deep sleep, as well as the cocktail of painkillers and lack of food in my stomach. I would obsessively check my steps. If I was clocking in slightly below the usual for that time of day, Princess Leia (my dog) would, once again, warily lift her head from the sofa and scoot under the throw blankets to avoid being taken on another walk, again. I had been doing yoga, stretches, chiropractic treatment, sports massage therapy, ice therapy, heat therapy (all of which is a huge privilege to be able to afford – the treatment, time and travel expenses), all based on my assumption that my poor, fat, useless and decrepit body was just unable to cope under the enormous strain of my 50 or so kilograms of, according to the BMI charts, 'additional' weight.

To find out that there was something, an actual reason I was in pain, was a relief. However, when I started to, as I think a lot of people do these days, Google obsessively about what causes gallstones, of course the first bullet point is: obesity.

Flashes of midwives laughing at me for wanting a water birth, to GPs snorting in derision when I asked if it was essential to weigh me today (when I was seeing them about a chest infection), or my elders commenting on my weight clouded all the other bullet points on that list.

Like point two: genetics – my sister having had her gallbladder removed just six months earlier. Or point three, that you are more likely to experience gallstones if you are assigned female at birth and have had children. So, even though out of the list of three possible 'reasons' I was in pain, and I qualified for all three of these 'risk factors', it was the fat part that I, and it would turn out, my healthcare professionals, just couldn't shake.

A few weeks later I am sitting down with a surgeon to discuss my treatment plan and he says that I should lose 30kg so they can operate. I won't sugar coat it – I crashed. Hard.

When the clinic first called to talk about my upcoming surgical consultation, they asked for my BMI. Not having scales in my house was less of a political or activist decision; it was a self-preservation thing. If the scales weren't there, I wouldn't have to know what they said. Then I wouldn't have to deal with the WeightWatchers or Slimming World of it all. But, more importantly, having listened at the feet of fat acceptance authors and influential beacons of knowledge and hope like Stephanie Yeboah[4] and Sofie Hagen[5] during my Audible-themed solitary dog walks, I cared less and less about what the scales declared me to be.

However, now I was being asked to confirm my BMI was under 45 so I could be treated at the smaller private clinic rather than having to go the big, longer wait-listed general hospital. Rather than face the scales in the shopping centre, with the imaginary (and non-imaginary) looks from folks ready to 'Step right up and see the incredible 20-stone person step on the scales, and maybe if we crane our necks, we can see what the numbers say and remark, "Glad that isn't me"', I opted for the cheapest next-day delivery digital scales I could find. Having confirmed my BMI was 42, I concluded that as I was under the threshold, I would be accepted for treatment at the clinic. I packaged the scales up and put them in the porch for the next day, when my dog walk would take me past the parcel store.

So, when I turned up to my appointment to be told I needed to lose around 30kg to be treated, I felt that immediate shame, rage and confusion that many a fat person knows all too well. They were uninterested in my multiple blood tests, urine, stool, ultrasound and stomach palpations confirming that, apart from the stones in my gallbladder, I was in good health. I remind myself frequently not to forget that within the last nine years alone, although this incredible, strong, warm and squishy body of mine had grown two babies, birthed

---

4   www.stephanieyeboah.com
5   www.sofiehagen.com

them, fed them, cared for my dying father, carried me across Glen Coe and up the fucking hills of Edinburgh Zoo (seriously, there should be a warning), along with living through a pandemic, through my grief, that I was still here, trying to eject these nasty little pebbles from my gallbladder, I was obviously 30kg too heavy to survive the keyhole surgery to give me my life back.

Want to know the worst bit about all of it? I fucking believed it. I was able to write off the bearing children and genetic elements so quickly and focus all the rage and blame for everything on my strong, fluffy, rounded, rolling, warm, fat body.

As I write this it is two weeks after that appointment, and despite trying to silence the voices of all the fatphobic comments I've ever heard, every snigger and every instance of my body and its strength and worthiness being questioned, I still hear those voices above the rest.

As I pulled on some of my leggings yesterday morning and I reached up to grab a shirt down, my leggings fell from my bellybutton to the floor. I grabbed the scales (that had remained in the porch parcelled for return for several weeks), tore off the inside-out return packaging and jumped on. I was 5kg down in two weeks. I hadn't been trying to lose weight, I hadn't been thinking of it; I had been thinking: my fucking stomach hurts all the time and if I eat, it comes out 20 minutes later, one end or the other.

By anyone's standards, apart from those touting crash diets and magic pills, 5kg is too much. Most folks will remind you of the 1–2lbs a week guideline. Yet the fatphobia crept in, over 25 years + of being diagnosed as fat at every turn, and it had built a common-sense-reflecting and impenetrable fortress in my mind. So much so that I am yet to call my doctor and add 'sudden and unexplained weight loss' to my growing list of symptoms.

After attending two more procedures to rule out other conditions that could explain my symptoms (that my straight-sized sister didn't have to have before her surgery – obviously), while waiting for the gastroenterologist, I once again noticed my clothes falling around me.

I retrieved the scales again from their packaging and now they totalled 12kg (just shy of two stones) less than my pre-surgical assessment weight. I had to factor in, of course, that I hadn't been able to eat for a few days here and there in the last few weeks because, while waiting for a gastroscopy or colonoscopy, you can't eat. Well, you can drink clear liquids and you have to drink the 'cleaner'. If you haven't had the pleasure, I will attempt to describe this. The closest substance in texture is gritty wallpaper paste. And if the texture wasn't enough to have you boking (retching), the taste will help: tropical. But not Lilt tropical, not delicious ice-cold can of Lilt on a hot day – oh no. This is chemically rotten, slight-hint-of-pineapple served in the style of lukewarm wallpaper paste. You're welcome...

So I got to the colonoscopy. Having been best friends with my toilet for the last 36 hours, having drunk only clear fluids (and still having to prepare food for my two children and remembering not to eat the ends of the carrots or testing their pasta was cooked by eating it!), I am reminded that I would need to wear dignity shorts.

The nurse taking care of me, Brenda,[6] was warm, reassuring and kind – exactly what I needed. I asked her, 'What is the largest size of dignity shorts you have? Usually the ones I am given don't fit, and it is uncomfortable and, frankly, embarrassing.' 'Don't worry', she quickly reassured me, 'we have very large sets, and I am sure you will fit.' Reassuring words said in the sweetest way still didn't convince me that all previous experiences of my rippling and jiggly butt and thighs ripping the paper dignity garments given to me in my lifetime would be different this time. However, when we went into the small recovery room to prepare, Brenda, the absolute diamond, unlocked the cupboard, showed me that they were arranged in descending size order, and said that she would excuse herself while I had a look through and got ready.

She didn't attempt to size me up or give me a pair; she simply showed me where they were kept, explained how I might navigate choosing, and left me to do the rest. This is the level of care, dignity

---

6   The name has been anonymized.

and respect I could get used to in healthcare settings. Brenda – don't go anywhere!

While I was slightly giddy from wearing dignity wear that wasn't bursting at the seams, and now being given medication to calm and relax me for the colonoscopy, Brenda leaned over, placed her hand on my shoulder and checked in by asking, 'Are you okay? AJ, are you comfortable?' I doubt that anyone, in a slightly chilly demountable hospital building wearing paper pants awaiting a camera to be navigated around their innards has ever answered with 'I'm having a lovely time!' My response was honest – I was having a lovely time! My retort was, of course, met with laughter, both nervous and genuine. Being treated like a human being and the service of having paper pants in your size can indeed turn the wallpaper paste starter and the main course 4-foot-long camera up your butt into a lovely time.

Even considering my combined days of nil by mouth before my gastroscopy and the aforementioned lovely time I had had at my colonoscopy, 12kg loss in a matter of weeks was concerning. It was even more concerning when it continued and I had to order new clothes. It continued to concern me more and more, especially when people kept approaching me and commenting on my body size. I assume that they themselves had also been indoctrinated into the diet and weight loss sphere. They had likely also been taught that fat = bad and dangerous, that they were paying me a compliment and that I would gush about how glad I was that my body was shrinking.

The first time it happened I was very taken aback. Having just collected my kids from school and carrying two backpacks, two lunch bags, one scooter and my last fucking nerve for the day already, a fellow parent on the school run crossed the road to approach me and said, 'You look *great*! You've lost *loads* of weight, right?' I barely got out a very apathetic 'Erm, yeah...' before she was gone after her own children. The second time, after having replayed the moment in my brain time and time again, was in the pharmacy, our lovely local pharmacy, where they give you three rings when your medicine is ready and remember your and your children's names. The person behind the counter said, 'Oh AJ, you've lost weight, right?' A simple

'Yes' I replied, in my best rehearsed neutral and matter-of-fact tone, while waiting for my medicine to be dispensed, thinking that my succinct response would be enough to quell any further attempts at discussion of my body, but no. 'Oh well, you look great! How did you do it? Have you been following a certain diet?' 'I've not been very well actually...' I replied sheepishly, not wanting to offend this lovely person who, again, I assume, considered their words to be flattering and complimentary. 'Well, you *must* feel better for it...do you?' 'For losing weight?' I clarified, and when they nodded enthusiastically, I was glad that the pharmacist appeared behind them to hand me my medicine so I could turn while giving my thanks and heading for the door. On the way home I repeated their words in my head, 'You *must* feel better for it...' 'You *must*...' What I had really wanted to say was, 'I've never been this poorly and for so long, so no, I don't feel better. This is the lowest my physical health has been, ever. I was healthier and happier when I was fatter.'

The third time was in the supermarket, and I happened upon an old family friend who was also on the prowl for a rotisserie chicken for dinner that evening. We stood around and chatted about the weather and how lovely my dad was and how sad she had been when she had been told about his passing, before she said, 'And Claire [made-up name of the family member they were actually talking about] said they had seen you and that you had lost weight, but she didn't say you had lost *this much*.' She even held out her arms to do her best emulation of a fat person. Still losing weight, I was about 17kg down (just over two-and-a-half stones) now, and in her defence, it was noticeable. Even folks I see fairly frequently had started to ask what diet I was trying. When the lovely man who I book to clear flotsam and jetsam from the gutters twice a year immediately greeted me as I opened my front door with his palms against his face and a '*Wow you've lost so much weight!*' I was so ready with my 'Please don't comment on my body shape or size' line. He was quick, however, to fire back staples from the big book of misogynistic comebacks, insisting that I should 'Lighten up, love' and 'learn to take a compliment'. If anyone knows a fat person who clears gutters in Essex, send them my way, will you?

I think I might try straight up ignoring people's comments on my body and start replying with something completely nonsensical next. 'Have you lost weight AJ?' 'Actually yes, we have had a new front door! Thanks for noticing!'

Or perhaps I should go in the other direction?

'You've lost weight! How did you do it?' 'Oh, like pretty much all fat people I have a long history of being treated poorly because of my body size, so I put off going to the doctor's for two years, plus my dad and nan died during that global pandemic and we couldn't go out for a walk for more than an hour at a time, once a day, and so I waited until my gallstones got stuck and I couldn't eat or drink anything without throwing it up or it firing out the other end within minutes of consuming it for two years...'

Maybe I should 'lighten up' and 'learn how to take a compliment'? Or maybe we should quit commenting on people's bodies changing. Unless it's a wicked new tattoo or something.

These experiences of people commenting on my body so openly always means I recall previous experiences of people commenting on my body. I remember a family member, assuming I was out of earshot, saying how I did look great, 'Especially for a big girl', on my wedding day. I also remember being knee high to a grasshopper in the back of my dad's brown Ford Capri with the tan roof (he was a bit of a sort) wearing a Pitsea Market special England kit for the Euro '6 campaign when that same family member turned in their passenger seat, looked me up and down, returned to my mum driving them to the train station and said, 'She is getting chubby now, you've got to stay on top of that.' Maybe it was just this family member...maybe not.

What about that time with the home economics teacher at school! As I was being fitted for my flying monkey costume for Shoeburyness High School's 2004 smash reprise of *The Wizard of Oz* they commented that they were going to have to go and buy more material because they 'hadn't counted on me being this...sturdy'. What about the music teacher, who thankfully didn't stay long, who said that I would struggle to acquire the required standard for my Grade 8 saxophone exam because my double chin and fat stomach would restrict my diaphragm and lip control. (Spoiler: I played that saxophone as well as many fat people before and after me.)

Or the theme park employee who loudly called across the queue to enquire what my weight was before allowing me to board the ride. Or the woman who, as I was sitting in a beer garden eating my meal deal lasagne and chips (same order as my size 10 friend sitting next to me), stopped en route to her friends waiting at another table to tell me, 'If you keep eating like that, you'll just keep on getting bigger.' Maybe it was just them...

Oh, but I remember that GP who laughed in my face when I asked about contraceptive options other than the injection because it messed with my mental health. He told me that losing weight would improve my mental health and then I could get other contraception options too! Or that other GP who said that my ankle probably wouldn't break again (this was the fourth time I had broken it, I think, all stemming from a sports injury, if you believe it – running for base in a game of Rounders as a teenager and my foot remaining stationary in a rabbit hole and the rest of me continuing onwards, then downwards), if I lost weight.

And I can't forget the midwife who sat back in her chair to laugh when I asked about a water birth. Followed quickly by, 'We would need to have a winch waiting for when you needed to get out; it's just not practical.' Oh, and what about the sonographer who all but cussed me while pushing the wand further and further into my tender pregnant stomach when they couldn't get the measurement they needed because 'it's just really frustrating when we can't get the right view past obese stomachs'.

How may my experience here translate to fatphobia in maternity and perinatal services, you ask? Well, if this service user, previously described as headstrong, lion-hearted, informed and experienced in navigating the 'isms' in a professional line of work can disregard giving my healthcare professional updates on my ongoing condition that is likely going to need surgery, can we imagine how, for some people, it seems impossible to disclose concerns or symptoms that worry them through fear of being diagnosed as fat?

Now having read my 'diagnosed as fat' comment a few times I realize I may have to explain. When fat folk are dismissed or even ridiculed for coming to a healthcare professional about their concerns or symptoms, we tuck that away. 'I always think to myself, okay, noted, arm pain is because I am fat. Or heavy periods, oh what do you know... fat. Broken arm? Fat!' Me, always.

There is already so much misinformation about when to seek medical care when pregnant, when spotting, lack of movement or the like, that adding another reason for folks to avoid seeking medical advice doesn't just seem cruel; it seems neglectful at best.

You can see how quickly women and birthing people who are told, or have it implied, that because they have a 'high' BMI they have developed gestational diabetes or pre-eclampsia, on top of being told that they cannot have a home birth or a water birth, can quickly lose faith in their bodies and the system that is meant to support service users in making informed decisions about their care and birth choices.

This also impacts the ability of service users to benefit from Midwifery Continuity of Carer (MCoC). In 2016 the Cochrane Review[7] confirmed what many had seen happening in their careers in birth: having continuity within your birthing team improves outcomes. Folks who received MCoC were less likely to experience preterm births or baby loss, or require an instrumental assisted birth. The study continues: 'Women who had midwife-led continuity models of care were more likely to experience spontaneous vaginal birth.' The authors summarize: 'This review suggests that women who received midwife-led continuity models of care were less likely to experience intervention and more likely to be satisfied with their care with at least comparable adverse outcomes for women or their infants than women who received other models of care.'

The article 'Pregnant and postpartum women's experiences of weight stigma in healthcare' in *BMC Pregnancy and Childbirth*[8] explains that service users who 'doctor shop' (those who frequently change

---

7   www.cochranelibrary.com/cdsr/doi/10.1002/14651858.CD004667.pub5/full, p.2.
8   https://bmcpregnancychildbirth.biomedcentral.com/articles/10.1186/s12884-020-03202-5

care providers) interrupt the MCoC model. For instance, in a sample of 20,000 patients, those with obesity had 52 per cent higher odds of doctor shopping compared to patients with a normal weight BMI. Additionally, in another article in *Obesity*, patients who were overweight and obese who engaged in doctor shopping had higher rates of emergency department visits, by 83–85 per cent.[9] I am sure that we can call the necessary and rightful search for informed and compassionate healthcare providers something less minimizing than 'shopping', though.

In the same review we are told about a study in America that showed that up to 74 per cent of medical students 'harboured implicit weight bias'.[10] In the UK, you might be forgiven for assuming the percentage of trainee healthcare professionals (HCPs) demonstrating significant levels of fatphobia would be less. But here comes the curve ball – it's higher, a lot higher – 98.6 per cent.[11] So less 'shopping' around with exacting standards of perfection and more searching for a healthcare provider outside of this 74 per cent. That's a 98.6 per cent majority that holds a bias about our fat bodies. Also, we undertake this search for good reason! *Weight stigma undermines the goal of treating obesity – which is weight loss.*[12] Weight stigma doesn't make people lose weight. It doesn't cure us of our 'affliction' or improve outcomes for mothers, parents or babies; quite the opposite.

A. Janet Tomiyama of the University of California describes weight stigma as 'vicious cycle' – a feedback loop wherein weight stigma begets weight gain.[13] Within Tomiyama's article the cyclic obesity/weight-based stigma (COBWEBS) model is described, how stigmatizing experiences lead to weigh gain, either through stress-induced cortisol secretion or mediated by coping attempts that promote eating and weight gain. So it is lose–lose. While weight stigma doesn't mean folks will lose weight, we do know that folks experiencing

9   https://doi.org/10.1002%2Foby.20189
10 http://doi.wiley.com/10.1002/oby.20687
11 https://pubmed.ncbi.nlm.nih.gov/23171227
12 https://bmcpregnancychildbirth.biomedcentral.com/articles/10.1186/s12884-020-03202-5
13 https://pubmed.ncbi.nlm.nih.gov/24997407

weight-stigmatizing healthcare are more likely to 'shop' around for a different healthcare provider. This could increase their isolation, as well as mean that they may not be able to benefit from MCoC. Additionally, those of us who are exposed to weight stigma throughout our lives, or pregnancies, are then caught in the 'cycle of weight stigma'. Then we return to our next appointment, possibly heavier, are weighed (which you can decline), and are then subject to more weight stigma, and so the cycle repeats.

Then, when you take into consideration that diets, largely, don't work,[14] we must wonder what benefits, if any, come from weight stigma? The goal of healthcare interactions is to benefit the service user, to pass on information and to improve their health conditions and/ or emotional state, right? I often glumly quip that a lot of HCPs seem to assume I don't know I am fat. [AQ] The frequency and strength of many assertions from HCPs throughout the years has only cemented the assumption I hold that they assume that I live unaware of my size, so unencumbered that it is their duty to inform me I am fat. And frequently.

The 'Dieting does not work, researchers report' article goes further. It states:

> you can initially lose 5 to 10 percent of your weight on any number of diets, but the weight comes back. We found that the majority of people regained all the weight, plus more. Sustained weight loss was found only in a small minority of participants, while complete weight regain was found in the majority. Diets do not lead to sustained weight loss, or health benefits for the majority of people.[15]

Traci Mann, Associate Professor at UCLA, and lead author, goes on to explain that most people in the study 'would have been better off not going on the diet at all. Their weight would be pretty much the

---

14   www.sciencedaily.com/releases/2007/04/070404162428.htm
15   https://newsroom.ucla.edu/releases/Dieting-Does-Not-Work-UCLA-Researchers-7832

same, and their bodies would not suffer the wear and tear from losing weight and gaining it all back."[16]

We need to be clear when we say diets don't work: they don't, but more accurately, as far as health is concerned, they don't improve outcomes in obesity-related concerns for fat folks.

Weight stigma from HCPs doesn't mean that people are more likely to lose weight (COBWEBS); even if people do diet, they are unlikely to maintain the weight loss. In fact, they are more likely to gain it back, plus some. We also have increased isolation, negative mental health impacts, deregistration or lack of engagement with HCP services, and more.

What does all this mean for fat, pregnant folk?

HCPs recommending dieting or weight loss during pregnancy, given its fixed time parameters and the negligible (if any) benefits – even if you are in the single-digit possibility of *successful* dieters – is more likely to cause weight gain than weight loss. It is also likely to disrupt your healthcare outside of your weight or BMI too. The very offer[17] of weight management services by HCPs can do more harm than good.

So what's the alternative? If HCPs can't speak about BMI and weight-related risks, then how are those HCPs able to pass on information to service users that will improve their outcomes? Consider the COBWEBS model again. There is an overwhelming likelihood that even bringing up BMI and weight management to fat folks in pregnancy will have a negative impact on them, it's unlikely that even if (in the UK) a fat person found one of the 1.4 per cent of the next generation of healthcare workers who don't hold fatphobia within themselves,[18] and they were in the 5 per cent of people for whom diets don't fail, that there would be anything other than slight improvements in health outcomes. Weighing this up against the harm that can be caused by weight stigma in healthcare, it seems risky to assume the current methods of informing fat service users of the increased

16 https://newsroom.ucla.edu/releases/Dieting-Does-Not-Work-UCLA-Researchers-7832
17 All treatments, scans, procedures, tests etc. should be offered on the merits of their benefits, risk and informed consent.
18 https://pubmed.ncbi.nlm.nih.gov/23171227

risk to them and their babies are working to improve outcomes for parents and babies alike.

Before we even get into the 'pregnancy is a great time to lose weight' bullshit, we must pause.

I want to ensure that the above has left its mark.

It is unlikely that losing weight, even when it works and sticks, will decrease risk or improve outcomes. Exposure to weight stigma and/or insisting that service users lose weight or diet in pregnancy is much more likely to have negative impacts on social, emotional and physical outcomes than positive impacts.

Being advised to lose weight in pregnancy isn't an uncommon occurrence for fat folks, but even a plateau of weight in pregnancy should, arguably, be considered a loss of weight. When you consider the weight of the necessary changes and additions to pregnant women and people's bodies (like the baby, placenta, increasing mass of the uterus as well as amniotic fluid, breast tissue growth etc.), maintaining weight from preconception or early pregnancy to the baby's birthday must mean a reduction in weight of the gestational parent has occurred. Your body is literally creating life. It doesn't need calorie deficits. It needs lush, fresh varieties of food groups that bring you joy. Movement that feels good and releases oxytocin would be great too!

This is much closer to the direction that NHS Highland has taken with their 'Healthy weight' document.[19] In this NHS Highland prioritizes improving the quality, variety and amount of food people eat. It also talks about eating in response to internal cues of hunger and fullness as well as recognizing emotional eating, having a social life, and doing physical activity that people enjoy. Furthermore, they make sure to include building good self-worth, self-care and body respect.

I include this final paragraph too: 'larger people are often stereotyped as not bothering about their health and given other negative characteristics. Everybody deserves respect, whatever their size, shape, fitness level, health status, eating patterns etc. Learning to look after

---

19 www.nhshighland.scot.nhs.uk/health-and-wellbeing/healthy-weight

yourself and protect yourself against these stereotypes may be difficult, but it is important.'[20]

Moving away from the blanket statement of fat = bad provides all folks, regardless of BMI, with the information needed to improve their wellbeing. From eating to hunger cues to moving your body in ways that you enjoy, NHS Highland manages to convey this information without the assumption that fat folks eat only fast food and never move, apart from to the fridge.

Fat folks do incredible things with their fat bodies. The bodies that societies not only hide but insist that we, too, also hide, hide that I like my body. My body is so strong. That's even worse than just being fat for some. Not only that you exist, but that you aren't actively trying to change that, to make yourself more acceptable?

My friend, who wished for me to anonymize their experience, perfectly demonstrates why this COBWEBS model, or continual feedback loop, is harmful.

I have a binge eating disorder and I weight cycle, regularly – my BMI has been between 20 and 35, so right across multiple brackets of BMI categories. I entered my first pregnancy with a BMI of under 30, and my second, I was over 30. The difference in treatment was bloody amazing. But I ended my first pregnancy with a weight higher than I started my second pregnancy. So I was very low weight to start with, and it shot up during pregnancy. Nobody noticed because I had already been weighed and my BMI recorded as it was at the time, and nothing more was said about it. I was experiencing symptoms of my binge eating disorder during pregnancy, which isn't good for you, but is especially negative for you during pregnancy and for the baby as well. Gaining that much weight so quickly in pregnancy is reason to be genuinely high risk and get further support, but because my BMI was taken at the start, and it was 'normal', no one seemed to care. In my second

---

20   https://tam.nhsh.scot/therapeutic-guidelines/therapeutic-guidelines/food-fluid-and-nutrition/healthy-weight/healthy-weight-health-improvement-guide

pregnancy the care from the NHS was just focused on my BMI. That is the reason I used an independent midwife; the NHS was not focusing on my care given my history of eating disorder, or my PTSD [post-traumatic stress disorder] from my previous birth, nothing about my previous traumatic caesarean birth, nothing about the fact that I had nerve damage from the epidural I was given – none of that was a factor. The NHS care was all about the fact that I was big.

The care that I received, as someone with a binge eating disorder, I think would have been enough to give someone with a dormant eating disorder an eating disorder. In my first pregnancy my eating was controlled, and my disorder was dormant. At my first appointment they insisted on weighing me, even when I offered to tell them my BMI as I already knew it and knew my weight, and it would be accurate to within a pound. They insisted, and that was the first time in eight years that I had stepped on any scales, and that is when my eating disorder reactivated. That is why I was so much heavier by the end of my pregnancy. The harm caused there by midwives not understanding actual psychiatric-diagnosed conditions such as eating disorders was massive.

Even outside of pregnancy care the lack of knowledge from HCPs on eating disorders is dangerous. At the start of 2020 I was experiencing persistent sinus infections. I tried treating myself, and they kept coming back, and then COVID-19 hit so it was about two years before I got in front of an ENT (ear, nose and throat) surgeon. Before she had asked me anything about my sinus infections or the like, she asked me if I had considered losing weight. I stopped her and said, 'If you look at my notes, you'll see I have a binge eating disorder. Please do not talk to me about weight loss.' But also, how many fat cells are inside nasal passages? I asked her this and she confirmed that there are none. But she still asked me five more times in that appointment alone if I would consider losing weight. To say to anyone who is AFAB [assigned female at birth] 'Have you considered losing weight?' is just ridiculous. Of course I have! The entire world has been telling me to lose weight my entire life. When she called for the follow-up appointment, the first thing she said wasn't 'How have you been?' or 'Are you still experiencing difficulty with sleep and struggling to breathe?' It was 'Have you lost any weight?'

Experiences of medical fatphobia or size bias are not exclusive to pregnancy. Even during what most people working in the field would agree is the most vulnerable time of women's and other pregnant people's lives – fat people experience fatphobia.

CHAPTER 2

Fat, Black and Pregnant

When thinking about the countless women and people whose stories I had heard on this subject, I knew I wanted to include Fiona Houston's words in this book. I first met Fiona during 2020 when I was working alongside other birth workers in the But Not Maternity campaign, and I followed Fiona on her Instagram account @FatBlackPregnant. Fiona had written some pieces surrounding her experience of being an older mother, a Black mother, and a fat mother. I asked Fiona if she would consider writing her story and contributing to this book. I knew that not only would it be moving and educational, but also that it would help humanize mothers and other fat, pregnant people.

Fiona Houston's experiences

I've been fat almost my whole life, so getting even fatter for a year really meant nothing to me at all. I just wanted to be a mum because, well, I knew I'd be good at it. But I also knew that if I ever got pregnant, my weight would be a huge focus.

Now there are definitely days where I'd like to push her back inside of me and pretend like she never happened (toddlers really are as hard as they say, in the best possible way). But ultimately, becoming a mum was a role that I genuinely knew that I'd be great at. It wasn't something that I'd always wanted – I'm not one of those people who had always dreamed of becoming a parent. It was meeting my husband that solidified a belief I'd been holding inside of me for a long time, a desire that I had never said out loud until Jack.

Before I became pregnant with my daughter, I miscarried at

around eight or nine weeks. When we had the positive test for that first baby, we were so excited. We told our parents straight away and we were bubbling with an excitement I'd only felt a handful of times before. Like the day I got married, or drinking in Trinidad, Cuba on our honeymoon, or on our third date when I told Jack I loved him for the first time (and meant it).

When I started bleeding and cramping, my first words to both Jack and the doctor who confirmed it the next day were 'I'm sorry.' I felt like such a failure. I'd failed our parents, I'd failed Jack, but more importantly, my body had failed that little foetus growing inside of me. And my fat body let it happen. My body was to blame. It had somehow betrayed me – how could it let my baby die and not let me know, for so long?

It feels so strange now to think that I punished myself so harshly at a time when what I needed most was kindness. I needed softness, but I didn't know how to find it. I needed somebody to blame. And so I hated myself. I refused to even give myself time to grieve and recover. Even though it took nearly four weeks for the miscarriage to complete, I went back to work long before I should have. I remember being in so much pain, sat on the sofa with my laptop open and trying to have a conversation with my mum without letting her know. I made an excuse about needing the toilet and I rushed upstairs and cried, biting into my arm to muffle the sound, holding cold water to my eyes to try and hide how flushed and awful I looked.

I was incredibly lucky to get pregnant again so quickly, I know that. It took maybe a month or a little over. I'm glad that we didn't put too much pressure on ourselves to make it happen, but that it happened quickly enough for my anxiety and fear not to have kicked in too much, preventing it from happening at all. However, it did mean that the distrust I had of my body was still raging inside of me.

I worried constantly that my body would fail me again. That I'd lose the baby and my body wouldn't let me know. Again.

One of the things I worried most about when I got pregnant (after my baby Ramona's health) was what would happen to my body.

Being fat and referred to as an 'obese, geriatric mother', I was terrified that my fatness would somehow harm my baby, that my body would become the villain in this love story that I was trying to create for myself and for my husband.

So, against my better judgement, I succumbed to all the additional tests that the hospital prescribed. I didn't question it when they insisted on weighing me at every appointment. I smiled at the nurse when she did a double take at the scales, incredulous at the number on the screen. I frowned but kept quiet when they seemed shocked that my GD [gestational diabetes] test was negative and when they insisted that I meet with the anaesthetist in advance of the birth to make sure she could find my spine. They didn't look at my back before making the appointment, didn't even lift my shirt for a cursory glance. So it was no surprise to me when my appointment with the anaesthetist lasted less than four minutes – she couldn't understand why they had sent me there. She lifted my shirt, pressed my spine and said, 'But there's no issue here.' I was just as frustrated as she was.

Looking back, the most frustrating experience was during the scans. I didn't mind the prodding, the being asked to move into lots of different positions. But the tutting, the looking irritated and throwing glances at colleagues; the words 'body habitus' on all the print-outs, with no explanation as to what that meant; I started dreading those appointments. They don't show you that on the television or in films: all you see are happy couples and 'perfect' bumps, the doctor finding the heartbeat almost instantly and grinning at the parents-to-be. Anytime you see a doctor struggle to find a heartbeat or to get a clear image, it's usually for a heart-breaking reason. So, every time they told me to lift my stomach, to roll onto my side, to walk around outside the room and come back, that terror came back, that feeling that my body was trying to fail me once again, that I'd betrayed the little person growing inside of me.

What I hadn't realized at the time was that every time we sat in a room and were essentially driven into decisions by fearmongering, my husband was just as terrified as I was. In fact, I would say, even more so. I had Ramona growing inside of me so I had something to anchor me, to push me through all the fear because I couldn't let her down.

I'm also pretty good at pushing aside any feeling that doesn't work for me in the moment (something learned in childhood that I can't shake, even after years of therapy). But Jack didn't have that. As the partner of the pregnant person, he could only watch as the two people he loved most in the world went through pregnancy and birth, something that every outlet told him was potentially lethal for fat women. In fact, Black women are four times more likely to die in childbirth so, as a fat and Black woman, the odds seemed firmly stacked against us. Every time a consultant told us how dangerous it would be for me to have a C-section as a fat person, it weighed him down. Every time they couldn't get a clear image of her, it weighed him down. When we had to do the prenatal screening twice, increasing the risk of miscarriage each time they took fluid from the amniotic sac, it weighed him down. And I didn't even know. He kept it all to himself out of fear of upsetting me. He let me rant and vent and cry at any given point, but he didn't want to add to my anxiety.

I had no idea the level of stress that all the negative advice and information had caused until I was taken into surgery for an emergency C-section. He got so quiet and looked at me with a slight panic in his eyes. After 30-something hours, I was happy to get her out of me, and I just couldn't understand why he looked so afraid. During surgery, I slipped in and out of consciousness – it felt like falling asleep. I don't know about you, but I'm one of those annoying people who will doze off while sitting up on the sofa and then get angry if you tell me I'm sleeping – I'll start talking complete rubbish, still basically asleep, but desperate to prove you wrong: 'The bicycle... I mean, the bicycle doesn't even have a mother, so how could it swim to the plane?' That's exactly what it felt like in surgery, like I was dozing off. But Jack wouldn't let me sleep, he kept shouting my name and I'd come round, chat complete rubbish and try to doze off again. I remember the people in the operating room telling him to let me sleep but he was adamant, never took his eyes off me.

Even once Ramona had been born and she was in his hands, he didn't want to leave. I had to insist that he take her and get out of the way. When they eventually rolled me out of surgery, he was sat there with Ramona in his hands, like he was holding a bowl of hot soup or a rugby ball. No smiles, no staring lovingly at the little beast in his hands. Just tears streaming down his face and his huge eyes, wide without his glasses. I will never forget the look on his face in that moment. Not just because I couldn't understand why he looked like that, but also because Jack never looks like that: terrified and just completely lost. He had to spend nearly an hour, sobbing alone with a newborn, convinced that he would never see me again. It was a long time after we left the hospital that he explained it to me: we had spent nine months being told that I was too fat for a C-section, that it would be dangerous for all involved. I now know that that is nonsense and, even when they were saying it, I wasn't really paying attention. But Jack was. He was paying close attention because they were talking about him potentially losing everything in one fell swoop. I don't think I'll ever forgive them for that, for what they put him through. Nobody should have to feel that way at a time that should be just full of joy.

What I've never understood about how they treat fat people in hospitals is, if it's so dangerous and awful for us to be pregnant and to have children, why don't they support us? Extra scans with people who don't respect us and telling us to join WeightWatchers isn't support. In fact, the special weight loss programme they insisted I join never actually materialized. I chased them multiple times and nobody ever got back to me. Being fat and pregnant is either so dangerous that they need to ram it down your throat at every opportunity, or it's not important enough to even return a phone call. It's one or the other, but it can't be both. Or at least it shouldn't be.

You'd think that the fatphobia would stop once you're in labour. It's a time of high emotion and everybody should have their eyes on the prize. I wanted to walk around and relax, and not labour in fear – I'm an anxious over-thinker whose mother lost a baby at eight-and-a-half months; I was already terrified. I had imagined walking around the room, dancing to my playlist and rubbing my belly, talking to the little baby making her way out of me. Before we went to the hospital we'd written her name on a pebble from Brighton beach, the same beach we'd raided for pebbles for our wedding tables, and I'd imagined holding it in one hand and Jack's hand in the other. I wanted to give birth on my knees and let gravity help me. I even wanted the pain. I wanted all of it. But they wouldn't let me. Because of my weight, they wanted me on my back and strapped to a monitor the entire time. I wanted to push back but I couldn't – what if they were right? I'd already been made to feel irresponsible for even getting pregnant while fat, so was I going to let my fatness ruin this, too? In labour, it's not just your heart that you're holding; it's your parents' and your partner's parents' and your partner's, someone you love more than yourself sometimes. So I did as they said and lay on a bed for 18+ hours. I found joy in hearing her heartbeat – it was so loud, it was like bathing in it. It didn't surprise me when things slowed right down. Maybe it would have been a long labour without their intervention, but we were doing good time at first, before they stopped me moving. And then it took hours and hours for full dilation. Well, I say full – I only made it to 9cm, and then they took me into surgery.

With everything I've read since giving birth, I'm convinced that all the medical interventions were the reason my labour stalled. From the sweep I didn't ask for, and the Pitocin (a synthetic oxytocin injection), to being made to lie still for so long. I'm also sure that I could have laboured for longer before needing surgery. But months of being told my weight would be an issue plus the expected emotional turmoil of a first-time experience made me malleable to, what I now believe, my own detriment.

Even once I was in surgery it felt like the people I was trusting to care for me had to really force themselves to show me any kindness. I'm a big girl, and that means I need higher amounts of drugs than someone smaller than me, someone of the standard size for whom most dosages are measured. By the time they took me into surgery, I had had two epidurals (they didn't tell me that it wears off if you don't regularly press the button) and a load of gas and air towards the end. I think they injected me with anaesthetic (it may have gone in through a drip, it's all a bit hazy now) to make me numb from the legs down. They expected it to work by the time we got to the operating room.

But it hadn't. They have this super-cold spray that they use on you to see if you're fully numb, and every single time they used it on me, I could feel it. They looked at each other, at me, back to each other, and then up at the consultant and the surgeons. They didn't believe me at all. Which makes no fucking sense because who on earth wants to be cut open when they can still feel everything?! Why would I lie?! So they had to give me more drugs, wait a few more minutes, and then check again. Which they did, and I could still feel it. They were incredulous – Jack had to insist that I wasn't lying (thank goodness I brought a white man into surgery with me!), and they did it again. Eventually I was numb, and everyone seemed a little confused and annoyed that they'd had to 'waste' 10 or 15 minutes waiting for my body to do as they wanted. Had they used common sense or taken the time to really consider me and my weight, they could have used the right dose in the first place and saved their precious time. Instead, they made me feel like there was something wrong with me.

Something else that Jack had to tell me after I left the operating room was that, during the procedure, my blood pressure kept crashing and machines were going crazy with beeps and bells. I still have no recollection of this, but perhaps that's why I kept dozing off. Once Jack left surgery, I remember going in and out of consciousness and looking up at the surgeons and/or consultants who were stood together, looking down at my stomach. I couldn't feel anything, but I watched them as they poked at my uterus, disgusted: 'Look at that. Flabby. I told you. Look!' They seemed horrified, not concerned. I was mortified and then passed out again, putting it out of my mind when I woke up because they were wheeling me out to Jack, with his shocked face and wide eyes. But when I remembered, I was so embarrassed. It made me feel like there was something wrong with me and that I should feel bad that they had had to deal with that. Nonsense. A little bit of research has told me that while 'flabby uterus' is a known phrase, it's also not something to joke about as it can cause real complications. What really stings is that they had that conversation while I was lying on the bed, entirely vulnerable and at their mercy. I felt like a tray of cat litter, something that nobody could be bothered to deal with.

They were the only people in the room, and I was entirely dependent on them to make sure I made it out of the room safely. In that fleeting moment, I felt entirely inconsequential; like I could slip away, and they wouldn't have noticed or really cared.

I mentioned that the 'flabby uterus' can cause complications or perhaps be indicative of further problems. I didn't know it at the time, but I was getting sick. Time is really fluid when you're in the hospital with a newborn, so it's hard to recall the details, three years later, and I can't remember the exact order of things. However, I do remember that I was looking forward to moving to a maternity ward. I really wanted a private room but ultimately was just happy to be away out of theatre. We were wheeled back to the ward I'd been on before Ramona was born. I had no idea why – the other women there were in early labour. I felt bad because they had to go through that with a squealing newborn in the same room, with just a thin curtain between us all. Because of COVID-19, that first night they told Jack to leave. He said 'yes', went to the toilet and then snuck back in and slept on the floor at the foot of my bed. And thank god he did because, despite having a C-section not six hours before, nobody came to help me during the night, not one person.

The next morning, Jack was cradling Ramona and I looked down at my thighs – they were huge. They're always huge, but now they were monstrous. I remember telling Jack that it looked like elephantiasis. I told a nurse or staff member and they looked at me like 'Isn't that just what your legs look like?' I insisted that 'I know what kind of fat I am, and this isn't it!' But they didn't care – nobody checked them or said, 'That's just normal water retention, don't worry.' Or, 'That's mental. We'll look into that straight away.' I decided to sit up and try to walk around (shuffle) to see if that would help the water drain. It didn't. So I tried to stop thinking about it – if they weren't worried, then why should I be? Jack was finally discovered and officially kicked out. I remember feeling tired and anxious, but also really wired: I had a baby! And she had a big, funny head and was perfect! I was figuring it out – nobody would come and help me get her out of the little cot, but I found a way to lift her without feeling like I was going to burst and without pulling out my catheter. And then it all got a bit weird.

That afternoon a consultant came to my curtain, frowning. I sat up and Ramona started fussing. The consultant looked at her clipboard, flipped some papers over and asked me, 'Do you actually want to get better?'

Now, when I say I had no idea what she was talking about, I mean it. Not only had I never seen her before, nobody had told me there was a problem. 'What do you mean? Is everything okay?'

'Your organs are failing. You have pre-eclampsia. You have sepsis. What is going on?'

I wish that I had felt stronger. I wish that I had been my normal self because she deserved the full force of Fiona rage. Since when has any one of those conditions been within a patient's control? Can you give yourself sepsis? When Dwight Schrute said in *The Office* (US) that he could raise and lower his blood pressure at will, were we the idiots for laughing at him?

This woman was glaring at me, angry, and fed up with me. I had no idea what she was talking about and had to cycle through terror, rage and concern for my newborn. If I have sepsis and fall into a coma, what will happen to Ramona, seeing as COVID-19 means nobody can come and see us? Ramona started to get really upset but I was feeling too shocked and weak to move. I asked the consultant to please help and give her to me. She looked at me and said, 'Most normal mothers would want to look after their child themselves. Don't you want to go home?'

She asked me about gestational diabetes and became the third or fourth person I had to tell that the tests had come back negative. She thought I was a fat, lazy, selfish witch who just wanted to luxuriate in a battered NHS hospital without my husband, family or anybody who would show me any kindness, never mind love me and my newborn.

I asked if Jack could please come back and she looked at me like I was an idiot. 'Yes, of course.'

I couldn't take it. They had made me feel so helpless, so stupid, just a disgusting beast that they didn't want to come close to. My daughter was crying and I couldn't physically move to her as quickly as I wanted to. They'd kicked out the one person who made me feel safe and then looked at me like I was crazy when I asked if he could come back. I sobbed. Honestly, I'm crying now just remembering how helpless I felt. I'm crying for someone who needed help, a hug, a smile.

The consultant looked so flustered, stepping back and her head pivoting in search of somebody to come help me. She disappeared without another glance. I ended up on intravenous antibiotics (I think – like I said, that time is a weird, blurry mess) and needed two bags of blood because I'd lost so much. I'll never forget having to text my family to tell them that I had sepsis and organ failure, but that they couldn't come to see me.

The next morning the consultant came back as part of the rounds that the Senior Consultant was doing with a group of doctors. She stood meekly behind him, offering a half smile and then looking down. The Senior Consultant said that I was recovering well and should hopefully be able to move to maternity from high risk (the first time I'd been told that I was on a high risk ward) that afternoon or evening. As they all turned to move to the next patient, I said very loudly, and while looking directly at the consultant, 'I'm so sorry about yesterday, I was just overwhelmed. You said all of those things and I was so tired and ill...' She quickly raised a hand, half a smile and a quick shake of the head, staring at the Senior Consultant the whole time, probably willing him not to turn his head and look back at us. He didn't.

Frustratingly, the shitty care continued into my time in the maternity ward – from staff refusing to help me move or to even push Ramona's cot closer to me, to searching for large absorbent pads the size of towels on which to change Ramona because nobody answered when I called for help, to someone coming in to tell me to hurry up and feed Ramona because her crying was disturbing everybody (at 2pm in the afternoon): it was a shit show.

If you're a parent, I'm sure you know the torture it is to need the toilet when you're trying to get a tiny baby to sleep. There is nothing more terrifying than putting a sleeping infant down – they're so sensitive to every movement and then, when you've got them down, it's like they can smell if you move too far away and wake up instantly. But I wasn't wearing a catheter anymore, I was desperate for a wee, and I hadn't had a shower in four days. I just needed eight minutes alone to fulfil these simple, basic, human needs. By some miracle, Ramona didn't even twitch when I gently pushed her little cot from the bed. She was silent and serene while I put my robe on and shuffled off of the bed. Not a peep came from her as I closed the curtain around her and made it to the toilet. I had a wee and then stood in silence: nothing. I stripped and turned the shower on; it was gross in there, but it was one of the best showers I've ever had, all 3.5 minutes of it. I turned the shower off and there it was: the tiny snarl of my little baby, alone and desperate for me to come back. I was soaking wet and my clothes were on the floor but I grabbed my robe and went to her, people giving me angry looks instead of offering to help. I closed the curtains behind me and soothed her. Once she was quiet, I went to get my clothes and came straight back. As I was pushing my arm into a sleep bra (I got them from Evans or maybe from Yours – they're fucking amazing, I still use them now!), someone swept back the curtain. My boob was hanging out and I had no idea what was going on. A staff member looked me up and down. 'Are you that baby's mother?'

'Yes.'

'Oh, okay. Must be. I saw how fat the baby was and wanted to see if the mother was fat too.'

Then she turned around, dragging the curtain closed behind her and disappeared back into hell, I guess. Again, I truly wish full-rage Fiona had shown up. Honestly, I'd probably be banned from that hospital for life.

My first night in maternity, Ramona started cluster feeding. It was some ridiculous time of night – after 2am – and Ramona had been feeding from me for hours. She'd feed for 15 minutes, come off and then scream almost instantly for more. My milk couldn't refill fast enough; I was crying and falling asleep while holding her because I hadn't been able to sleep for more than maybe two hours in so long. I'd been warned about cluster feeding, but there is nothing that could have prepared me for that. I think, even now, that was the hardest experience for me of the first year of her life. I remember dozing off and she rolled down my thigh, the feel of her weight on my leg waking me just in time to catch her. I was beside myself; I thought I was losing my mind. I pressed the button so many times, desperate for someone to come. I just wanted someone to know that if I dropped her, it wasn't my fault. It wasn't intentional, please don't hate me. But nobody came. And then there she was. Out of nowhere came a ward sister – she walked towards me, smiling. She was an older Black woman, with neat black hair.

'What's going on here, mum?'

I couldn't open my eyes properly, they were so swollen from crying, and I was so tired. But I could see her smile. She was rubbing sanitizer into her hands, shoulders strong and a soft but authoritative expression. My family are from the Caribbean and so I had grown up with older Black women around me. They were rarely a source of comfort. Even the ones who truly love you so fiercely are often the most critical, the ones who will tell you that they think your make-up or outfit looks ridiculous, the ones who will tell you you're too fat, too rude, too soft for having therapy or taking medication. If you have immigrant elders in your family, then all this may sound very familiar. This woman, who appeared out of the darkness, smiling and in charge, had the same warm lilt as my grandmother, but she saw my weakness and didn't judge me. She came right up to the bed – the closest anybody had got to me for days – and looked down at me and Ramona. I told her that I thought Ramona was broken, that I had broken her somehow; that I was so tired I couldn't breathe. That I was entirely lost. She told me not to be silly and to hold Ramona to my breast. She actually picked Ramona up and put her against me, gently lifted my hand and put it so that I was holding Ramona to me. It's just occurring to me now that she was the first person to touch Ramona who wasn't me or Jack. And then she disappeared to a cupboard, returning with an armful of pillows. She packed pillows into the bed behind Ramona and along both sides of the bed, so that neither one of us could move. I relaxed my arm and Ramona stayed nestled against me. I was free to sleep if I needed to, without fear.

It was the most incredible sense of relief and I slept for nearly four hours. I woke up to a sleeping Ramona and a soft light coming in through the curtains.

Maybe 20 years ago, while out shopping with my mum she turned to me, with the craziest look in her eyes; she was just hyper out of nowhere. I asked her what was happening and she just squeezed my hand and followed a woman into a card shop. When I caught up with her, she was talking to the woman with tears in her eyes. 'You delivered all three of my girls. You were so kind to me when I had to deliver my eldest; she was stillborn at eight-and-a-half months. I've never forgotten you – I was going to give my second daughter your name as a middle name. I'll never forget you.' I did not understand it at the time – why on earth would you remember someone who was just there, doing their job? After that night with Ramona, I get it now.

In the fog of birth and that time in hospital, there are so many broken fragments of moments, good and bad: listening to my favourite songs by candlelight while looking out at the sunset, falling in and out of consciousness on the operating table, sitting alone and bleeding with a screaming baby in my arms and sobbing. But that night, with the ward sister coming to keep me and Ramona safe, is something I hope to keep with me forever. I'm broken hearted that I don't know her name – I didn't see her again after that night. My foggy brain worried that I'd made it up, but the nine pillows in the bed put that thought out of my head pretty quickly. I asked about her but I couldn't get a straight answer from anybody, and the normal service of being made to feel like an inconsiderate drain on resources resumed.

I do sometimes wonder how bad my time in hospital would have been if not for COVID-19. Ramona was born the day lockdown started and I was in hospital for a week; I saw first hand the confusion and terror that the staff felt. The rules about who could be in the hospital kept changing, and I don't doubt they were scared to get too close to anybody. I'm sure the consultant who blamed me for my organ failure was operating under a lot of stress. However, so much of what upsets me now, three years later, is the way they looked at me, the assumptions they made about me because of my body (and my race), and how they made me feel totally worthless. That wasn't COVID-19. That was a complete disrespect and disregard for fat bodies and our experiences. I often wonder what it would have been like to experience all of that while depressed. I have an extensive mental health history, a lot of which was rooted in pure hatred of myself and my body. To have been made to feel like I was disgusting, undeserving of care and entirely disposable, at a time when the all-consuming weight of being the only person present to care for a newborn, feels criminal. Whether it was intentional abuse or subconscious bias towards people who look like me (fat, Black and over 30), they have a duty of care, perhaps even more so during a fucking pandemic, to help the vulnerable feel supported. It felt like they had kicked me out of a plane without a parachute and spat on me when I reached out for help. Had I been in a vulnerable mental state, I hate to think what could have happened to Ramona.

I just read that back and I'm speaking as if I didn't have mental health relapses while I was there. I really did. There were moments where Ramona was sobbing and I was crying so hard that I bit on my arm so that she couldn't hear me. I didn't want her to feel more scared than she already did. I've never felt so alone in my life.

But from that loneliness came a feeling of love and dedication and protection for Ramona that I'm not sure would have been there without that trauma. I mean, of course it would have come at some point. But I had no time to recover, nobody with me to give me a breather, and surrounded by healthcare professionals who made me feel unsafe. The only absolute that I knew during that time was that Ramona needed me. I held her in my arms, stroked her face, kissed and smelled her head, and just wanted so desperately to fight for her. I had to keep her safe for all of the people who were waiting for us, climbing the walls waiting to meet her. She wasn't just the centre of my world: she *was* the world. I started to rely on this fat, Black body to keep us both safe: Ramona safe from everybody else and me safe from my depression and hopelessness. Sometimes it felt like I was watching my body do things from afar, like I was trapped inside a tiny version of myself, sitting on my big self's shoulder; silent and overwhelmed. My body kept us both alive, answered texts from family, filmed Ramona so that Jack didn't miss anything she did (which was nothing really, because she was no more than four days old, but you couldn't have convinced me of that at the time!).

And my body continued to impress me. I got to know 'Her' in a way I never had before. She was so strong and brought Ramona so much comfort. She produced an abundance of milk so that no amount of cluster feeding would defeat Her again, something that I now think was in response to Ramona's undiagnosed tongue-tie. It didn't matter that the health visitor refused to come and see us and stopped answering my calls, or that nobody would help us with her tummy troubles for three months; my body got us through it. I even fell in love with the weird, saggy belly, finding comfort in stroking it while trying to fall asleep.

I found a strength and belief in my body that I had never had before. I regained the trust and found a faith that it would see us through anything. I will never lose that again, and that's all because I survived. And as Ramona grows and stops needing me to survive, I will never forget what my body did for us, what *I* did. This is the body that my daughter will remember holding her, feeding her, pushing her on the swing. This is the body that she rode around the living room like a bucking bronco and that chased her around the park. This body is her mother, and her mother is a fat old woman. And there's nothing more powerful than that.

CHAPTER 3

Conception

To quote Julie Andrews, let's start at the very beginning, a very good place to start.

Having never used assisted conception services myself, the briefest of peeks into the requirements and stories of restrictions in access on communities such as Big Birthas showed me exactly what I assumed was happening. A BMI of 30+ = blanket exclusion.

This must be backed up in many peer-reviewed studies and systematic reviews that prove that BMI 30+ means you are less likely to conceive, purely because of your BMI, right?

A systematic review on the effect of overweight and obesity in women undergoing assisted reproductive techniques concluded that there was insufficient evidence to link high BMI with reduced live birth rates (Maheshwari *et al.*, 2007). Compared with women with BMI>30 kg/m², the odds of pregnancy in women with BMI<30 kg/m² were 1.16 [95%: confidence interval (CI) 0.95, 1.43] (Maheshwari *et al.*, 2007). In women, with BMI<25 kg/m², the odds of pregnancy per woman were 1.24 (95% CI: 1.02, 1.50) and per cycle, 0.99 (95% CI: 0.88, 1.12) in comparison with women with BMI≥25 kg/m². This meta-analysis, based on aggregated observational data, was unable to adjust for key confounders such as age, duration of infertility and previous pregnancy. Given the uncertainty surrounding the interpretation of these results, it is difficult to conclude that there is a causal relationship between obesity and live birth rates following IVF and identify a threshold BMI above which success rates are so low (or complication rates are so high) that treatment should be withheld. The debate is further enlivened by results from a recent study showing that obese patients (BMI>30 kg/m²) who respond normally to ovarian stimulation have conception rates which are no lower than those with a BMI<30 kg/m² (Orvieto *et al.*, 2009).[1]

Also in the same review…

absolute risks in women who are overweight or obese class I (BMI<35 kg/m²) are low (Callaway *et al.*, 2006; Abenhaim *et al.*, 2007; Bhattacharya *et al.*, 2007) and do not justify the cut off values currently recommended in the UK, Hong Kong and New Zealand to restrict access to IVF.[2]

Maybe it's about cost…?

It has been argued that providing fertility treatment to overweight and obese women is not cost effective due to poor chances of success, higher risks of pregnancy loss and perinatal complications (Gillet *et al.*, 2006). Yet, the literature on the costs of fertility treatment, antenatal and peripartum care in obese women is sparse. A recent study failed to show any significant differences in costs per live birth following ART in overweight and obese women compared with women with normal BMI (Maheshwari *et al.*, 2009).[3]

Bring it home with the conclusion then…

Overweight and obesity is common in women of reproductive age, many of whom are choosing to delay childbearing thus creating a need to balance the detrimental effects of age versus BMI on fertility and perinatal outcomes. Robust data showing an association between BMI and live birth in subfertile women are lacking. Available evidence

---

1   https://academic.oup.com/humrep/article/25/4/815/700269, p.815.
2   https://academic.oup.com/humrep/article/25/4/815/700269, p.816.
3   https://academic.oup.com/humrep/article/25/4/815/700269, p.817.

suggests that age has a stronger negative impact on fertility and pregnancy outcomes. There is insufficient evidence, at present, to deny women fertility treatment on grounds of BMI given the relatively poor success rates of most weight loss regimens and discriminatory nature of such a policy against half the female population of many countries. Weight loss should be encouraged wherever possible and preconception counselling offered. However, the gain associated with weight loss in older women needs to be balanced against much steeper loss in fertility with age. In a population where over half of all women are overweight, it can be argued that is unfair to insist on their adherence to an outdated measure of normality, and simplistic to exclude them from fertility treatment.[4]

Well, *quelle surprise* – insufficient data to conclusively back a link between BMI 30+ and infertility. If, like me, you have limited or no experience of conception services, fear not. We are lucky enough to have Nicola Salmon, author of *Fat and Fertile*,[5] to help guide us through the difficulties that fat folks may experience in seeking fat-competent or even fat-neutral care. If you are fat and in the process of conceiving, I can't recommend Nicola's book highly enough. *Fat and Fertile* should be essential reading for anyone working with hopeful mothers and parents. Not only are we just as worthy as any other people, but a lot of the information we have been given about the risks of being fat isn't factual. It hasn't taken into consideration comorbidities, and it comes with a healthy dose of implicit weight bias.

I sat down with her (virtually, obvs) to talk about all things conception and fat!

Interview with Nicola Salmon

AJ: I had a wee scan of your book again in preparation for sitting down with you today, and I circled it the first time I read it, and

---

4   https://academic.oup.com/humrep/article/25/4/815/700269, p.818.
5   https://nicolasalmon.co.uk/fat-and-fertile-book

for want of a pen this time would have circled this question again, because I think it's a real doozy! 'What would happen if you stayed exactly as you are?' I think it sets off this, like, light bulb moment with a fair little dusting of panic at the same time because nearly all interactions I have had with HCPs about my health or wellbeing have focused on how I could be less. So, when we ask that question regarding conception services, that must be a terrifying prospect for fat women and people. Staying the same means being denied access to conception services in some trusts.

So I want to ask you most about that question. I mean, I think we could do a whole hour just on that question because I think it's a great fucking question.

Nicola: Easily an hour! When I wrote the book, that question came from a place of 'What if I just stopped hating my body? What if I could never, ever, do anything to change my body? What if all that control is taken from me?' There is so much responsibility placed on us to change our bodies to access care, to get referrals or operations. So when I wrote that question, I was trying to take that responsibility for change away from myself. Of course, we are all responsible for ourselves, but the question flips the responsibility for lack of access or support back to where it belongs – with the people who are restricting access, based on not very much at all. We have this culture that is driven by change, that's capitalism. Get a bigger house, a faster car, a thinner and therefore better body, right? What if the aim of our lives was just to happily exist, how we are and where we are? Searching for things that bring us happiness and joy without this undercurrent of better, faster, thinner?

So really the question is, are we happy now? Do we want to change it? Do we need to change it?

AJ: Yes, and it speaks to the realization that this internalized fatphobia or internalized size bias is this heavy fucking thing that a lot of fat folks are carrying around. What happens if we put that down? What are our hands and minds freer to see, do and experience now?

Nicola: Hmmm...yes!

AJ: And fat people put off so many things like holidays or experiences, travels, work, sex, relationships, moving their body for the sheer fucking joy of it, and what if we just did all those things while we were fat?

Nicola: The things we miss out on, and the *money* we waste, while we are waiting for or while we are in pursuit of thinness.

AJ: It poses that question of 'Can we be, not even happy but neutral enough about ourselves to be happy right here and now?'

Nicola: Mmmm...yes, and what you said before about the weight of the fatphobia. I remember the time that I stopped weighing myself and dieting and the weight of centring thinness, letting go of the ideal body shape or size. Being able to exist without the weight of all of that on my mental health and my physical health. The way we restrict food, the way we restrict movement and how we can berate ourselves for gaining weight or even maintaining weight. Or even not losing weight fast enough. Just put it down – it's too heavy to carry forever.

AJ: I hear you! Another thing I love about your book is that the myth busting starts almost immediately. There are so many myths about BMI and conception, so it is fabulous that, front and centre, these myths are busted.

Nicola: The headline is that your BMI says nothing about your fertility. So many people put off starting or growing their families in the pursuit of weight loss, because we are told that fat people can't conceive. It's also about the internal ethical debate that happens for many fat people. Thinking or saying something along the lines of 'Should I get pregnant at this size because I am going to be at a higher risk of this or that?' So, giving people that information up front to enable them to change that narrative and say, 'Well, I can start or grow my family at my size because BMI isn't linked to fertility or more worth.'

AJ: Because even on the NHS website it actually says 'being a healthy weight', which the NHS states on other documents is a BMI of between 19 and 30, right?

Nicola: Yeah, it's everywhere.

AJ: So that comes back to your great question... 'What happens if we stay the same?' This is going to have a knock-on effect on people's lives; their whole life plan can be blocked because of these criteria.

Nicola: Absolutely, because we cannot control our weight. Weight is unmodifiable. We can, in the short term, reduce it by controlling calorie intake. We know that 95 per cent of the time it's only for a short window and we are likely to regain that weight, plus more! We cannot modify our weight. HCPs (by and large) seem in denial about this. And they will say the same things over and over, how 'If you lose weight [insert ailment here] won't be a problem anymore.'

AJ: Or these infuriating, condescending and oversimplifications of 'eat less, move more'.

Nicola: [faux vomit noise]

AJ: Right? Because it all has the same meaning. Once you boil it down, distil it all, it's just fat = bad all over again.

Nicola: Yes, that is the foundation of it, yes.

AJ: The foundation of everything bad, right? Bad access, bad health, bad parenting, bad visibility, bad self-worth, bad fertility? Fat = bad.
    Without expecting you to solve the whole world's fatphobia, then, where does this come from? Fat = bad regarding fertility specifically? Because it wasn't always that way. We see fatness celebrated and carved into precious metals in First Nation and Indigenous communities and ancient civilizations, right?

Nicola: So fatphobia is inherently racist. White European colonization sought to elevate whiteness as superior to Black, Brown, Indigenous and First Nation peoples. One of the ways to do that is to demonize certain body shapes and types. Demonizing certain aspects of Indigenous, Black and Brown bodies is an arm of white supremacy. Great books on that subject to read are: Da'Shaun L. Harrison's *Belly of the Beast* and Sabrina Strings' *Fearing the Black Body*. It's one of the ways that colonizers sought to elevate themselves above Indigenous, First Nation, Black and Brown people. It was health insurance companies that first started using BMI as a means for categorizing people as 'high risk'.

AJ: And, as I know you know, and we have already covered in the first pages of the book, BMI is biased and unreliable in measuring health.[6]

Nicola: It makes zero sense, and the 'cut-off points' have been changed previously, so overnight,' people are now obese? Did their risk change? Did their bodies change?

AJ: This is another common barrier for folks in maternity or perinatal services too. At one trust their 'cut-off' for access to a maternity unit or midwifery-led unit might be 35, but in another it is 30. Or some trusts and even some HCPs will be more 'lenient' than others, and while I hear you, so much is a postcode lottery in the NHS and there isn't an endless amount of funding... Can it still be justified to restrict fat folks' access to fertility services based on an outdated, inaccurate equation from hundreds of years ago used to determine the average weight of a population of white, European, non-disabled, cisgender men?

Nicola: No, it's not.

---

6   www.ncbi.nlm.nih.gov/pmc/articles/PMC4890841
7   www.ncbi.nlm.nih.gov/pmc/articles/PMC4890841

AJ: So theoretically, then, a hopeful mother who has a BMI of 33, for example. She may be told or feel that her only option to access fertility treatment is to crash diet. We know that diets don't work;[8] more and more studies and reviews are showing us that BMI reduction doesn't improve fertility,[9] and we know the dangers of crash dieting[10]... make it make sense!

Nicola: One of the reasons is a lot of the research looks at people as two distinct groups: people in bigger bodies, and people who are in smaller bodies. What they are assuming is that people who are smaller bodied are the same as people who were in bigger bodies and have lost the weight. They assume that someone who has always had a BMI of around 25 is the same as someone who had a BMI of 40 and lost weight to now have a BMI of 25. We know that doesn't make these two people the same. We know the effects that dieting has on you physically, as well as psychologically. We know that people are more likely to weigh more than when they started dieting. Or they drop a lot, then gain a bit back, then drop more, then gain a lot back – this is called 'weight cycling'.

When your body goes through this process of weight cycling it has a negative impact on your body, on your stress or cortisone levels, your metabolism, and it impacts your hormone levels, it affects how all your body works. We know from so many studies that when we go on an extreme calorific reduction diet our body doesn't say, 'Oh, okay, I know I am safe, and this is a diet.' It says, '*Fuck*, I am in danger! I might starve!' The body enters a stress state, and it stores fat and reduces its metabolism down so it burns as little as possible to keep fat reserves up because danger is coming, and we might have to run away! The body tells us, 'I need sugar, I need high-calorie food, now!' so that we can survive this danger or this famine. We are hardwired, for good reason, to hunker down, eat, conserve, and get ready for what is coming. Is it any wonder that if people manage to restrict

---

8   www.ncbi.nlm.nih.gov/pmc/articles/PMC4890841
9   www.sciencedaily.com/releases/2022/03/220314105639.htm
10   www.obesityaction.org/resources/the-risks-of-the-crash-diet

their calories enough to get these huge weight losses so quickly that their bodies are shutting down non-essential processes like ovulation? Our reproductive system shuts down because our body reasons, 'It is not safe to have a baby right now because I don't have enough food, I am not safe.'

Of course, people are going to keep going on these extreme diets because they are prescribed to them. They are told, 'Your BMI matters and time matters in fertility treatment', which is basically saying, 'Lose as much as you can as quickly as you can.' This can have a devastating effect on fertility.

AJ: So then, for fat folks who are starting their fertility journey, or folks who have been denied access to fertility services based on BMI alone...what, if anything, can we say to them?

Nicola: The first thing I always say is 'put the blame where it belongs', which is with the system and not with yourself. That can give people a sense of relief from the internalized and external shame that we feel as fat people. Unfortunately, there are no legal protections on access regarding size in the UK. There isn't any legal footing to fight these barriers with the NHS. I don't know of any trust that has a BMI limit higher than 30 (for access to fertility treatments). The reason is that we deem it acceptable to deny treatments to folks in bigger bodies. If our culture found that unacceptable, to restrict access to healthcare based on size, there wouldn't be a BMI cut-off. It's also based on money, finding a way to reduce the amount of people on waiting lists and the cost of running these services; they can cut around 30 per cent of their service user pool by excluding folks with a BMI of over 30."

In terms of what folks can do, they can put forward their case to individuals within the system or request reconsideration, follow complaints procedures etc. The UN (United Nations) does state:

11   https://commonslibrary.parliament.uk/research-briefings/sn03336

reproductive rights rest on the recognition of the basic right of all couples and individuals to decide freely and responsibly the number, spacing and timing of their children and to have the information and means to do so, and the right to attain the highest standard of sexual and reproductive health. They also include the right of all to make decisions concerning reproduction free of discrimination, coercion, and violence.[12]

Even though our basic human rights should mean that our reproductive rights are protected, it's a lot of onus to put on fat folks to advocate for their basic human rights. And unfortunately, not a lot of people will find themselves in a position to be able to fight that. Going through fertility treatment is an extremely vulnerable time for all folks, and it's no wonder that fat folks, who are likely to have experienced fat bias in healthcare before, aren't equipped with the resources and strength to fight the system that requires them to justify why they aren't any less worthy because they are in a bigger body.

So, you are between a rock and a hard place. Either go down the weight loss route that doesn't work in 95 per cent of the cases, and even where it does it could have a detrimental effect on your fertility. If you are able, you could access private healthcare in the UK, but even then, a lot of them have a BMI limit of 40 or more, and more clinics are reducing those limits too. Things are a bit better on the European continent – in Greece, Turkey and Czechia – where their BMI limits are more malleable. But people shouldn't have to take a month off their entire lives to fly thousands of miles to access the treatment they would have got for free if they weighed less. It is completely unacceptable that people are put into the position where they really don't have any choice but to accept that their reproductive rights aren't worth as much because of their BMI.

---

12 UN International Conference on Population and Development 'Programme of Action of the International Conference on Population and Development' para. 7.3. https://www.unfpa.org/publications/international-conference-population-and-development-programme-action

AJ: It's not giving humanizing, individualized healthcare vibes to me, right? Respect for autonomy and justice are supposed to be part of the ethical foundations of healthcare, and it's serving fat = bad over ethical or autonomous.

Nicola: It's wild. BMI 30 is a low limit, and it affects, like, a third of people who want or need access to fertility services.

AJ: We must presume that HCPs are aware of the same studies we are, that we found doing light research and Googling for a book about being fat, and why that sucks, right?

Nicola: Well, you'd hope!

AJ: Right? And that we know the majority of fat people have a 'normal' pregnancy and birth – we know that most fat people have a straight-forward pregnancy and birth and have healthy babies.[13]

Nicola: Right.

AJ: And interestingly, at the start of our chat, you said 'higher risk' rather than 'high risk'. Which I think is a very important distinction. 'High' and 'higher' have very different meanings. 'High risk' sounds like it is likely to happen. It sounds like it's more likely to happen than not to happen.

Nicola: And when you look at the studies and reviews, only about a third of them show there is a link between baby loss and BMI. A third showed there was a correlation, which doesn't equal causation, a third showed insignificant correlation and a third showed there was some correlation – off the back of papers and reviews like this they make sweeping statements that say there is a direct link with BMI and baby loss. It's barbarically fatphobic to do this.

---

13   www.rcog.org.uk/for-the-public/browse-all-patient-information-leaflets/being-overweight-in-pregnancy-and-after-birth-patient-information-leaflet

AJ: Is that why so much of your book is dedicated to unlearning this internalized fatphobia, then? Because when HCPs say to someone, 'You are high risk to have a miscarriage because of your BMI', and then if they experience loss, it's no wonder that we turn that blame and guilt onto ourselves. It is almost like we must confront the elephant in the room first, this internalized fatphobia and medical size bias.

Nicola: If someone wants to get pregnant and they still believe fat = bad, then they will do everything they can to stop themselves falling pregnant. If you believe that it would be really dangerous for you to be pregnant in your fat body, then you are more likely to procrastinate going to the doctor, you are more likely to do things that aren't in your best interest (like crash dieting) because you think that is safer than getting pregnant as you are. (What happens if you stay equal as you are now?) It is totally understandable that people hold this belief because it is drummed into us over and over again that fat = bad in regard to health and many other aspects. It's not fat folks' fault for thinking that, because we have grown up in a society and culture that tells us that fat is risk, fat is bad, fat is harmful. It is understandable that folks believe it is dangerous for them to be pregnant. Unlearning this and getting to a place where we believe in our bodies and feel safe being pregnant while fat isn't easy while we live in a society that continually tells us it's unsafe. We will continue to think that we aren't worthy of treatment, access, funding and humanizing care because we're told it is not safe.

AJ: That is a common theme among fat folks, that sense of unworthiness. Because society tells us we aren't worthy, continually. Unpicking that is scary because we then have to reframe all these previous and current experiences of being denied access; referrals or funding etc. were based on inconclusive or false pretences. And that maybe I wasn't being cared for by people who, consciously or unconsciously, thought of me as being as worthy as others because I live in a bigger body.

Nicola: You have to rewrite your past, and that is scary.

AJ: What do HCPs need to hear, then?

Nicola: Question everything. One HCP isn't going to change the world and bring down fat bias in healthcare, but you can question it. You can ask why we have this BMI cut-off for the birthing unit, for example. You can ask these questions of your superiors. You can call in colleagues about the way they talk to fat service users or what they write in our notes. The level of dehumanizing language that fat folks hear and have recorded about them is shocking. Having it recorded in your notes 'We couldn't get all the measurements we needed on the ultrasound because patient is fat' – is that okay? Is that acceptable?

AJ: Maternal habitus,[14] right?

Nicola: The thing is, if you go to a different sonographer, with the same or different equipment, you'll get a different measurement. And it's not just about the type of fat that obscures the ultrasound waves; it's because of the equipment and the training that the HCP has had. We can do so much better for fat people. HCPs need to have training on how to talk to fat people about their bodies. HCPs need to have training even in how to touch fat people's bodies. If maternal habitus is the reason that means that the type of fat this person has obscures the ultrasound, pulling at our skin and digging the wand in and twisting it round isn't going to change that. It just hurts and demeans us; it just increases the likelihood of us not wanting to have any more scans or go to any appointments because all they do is poke and prod at me, call me fat, write on my notes that I am fat and say that they can't help me because I am fat – why should I bother going back?

Question everything and question yourself. There is a great fat bias test[15] that you can do on the Harvard website. We are all fatphobic and we all have fatphobia and size bias within us because that's the

---

14 The physique or body build of the mother.
15 https://app-prod-03.implicit.harvard.edu/implicit/takeatest.html

result when we live in a society that is fatphobic. It is our responsibility to recognize and unlearn these biases.

AJ: And it's not like it's just a few HCPs who harbour size bias, right? It's nearly all of them – 98.6 per cent of trainee dietitians, nutritionists, nurses and doctors demonstrated significant levels of fatphobia.[16]

Nicola: Because it's built into the medical system, and it's built into our society. Look at children's books or Disney films – the heroes are thin and the baddies are fat.

AJ: Oh, and the villains are queer washed too. Think of the villains who are queer and fat coded. Ultimate example: Ursula. Fat and queer coded. Although now I'm thinking, Scar is thin and queer coded. Jafar is thin and queer coded. Now we've just gone off on one on Disney villains, ha ha!

Nicola: Even just the Mr Men books – my children love the Mr Men series, but look at Mr Greedy, Mr Lazy, Little Miss Boring, Little Miss Bossy and then look at Mr Awesome, Mr Cool, Little Miss Neat, Little Miss Somersault – it's coded from such a young age.

AJ: Even when I was looking for books about fat birth and my competitive title analysis the stark difference in book covers was remarkable. From yours, which has beautiful imagery, and *Fat Birth* by Michelle Mayefske compared to, well, I am not going to name them, but other 'plus size birth books' with headless fat people or just fat stomachs-covered books. Where else do we see the 'happy to be fat' representation?

Nicola: It's just not there. It is so absent in all aspects, but particularly in pregnancy. Perpetuating that ideal of 'doesn't even look pregnant' is harmful.

---

16 https://pubmed.ncbi.nlm.nih.gov/23171227

AJ: It's harmful for all folks; even for straight-sized folks it's harmful. The root cause, as it often is, is misogyny, framing women's clothing as plus size and men's clothing as big and tall, for example.

Nicola: It is the ultimate way to oppress people, right? Make them so concerned about the way they look or the way their bodies are perceived by others, so they don't have the power, energy or time to fight anything else.

Another way it shows up in medical settings is this reluctance for anaesthesia. It's presented as so dangerous for fat people to have anaesthesia, but they will recommend bariatric surgery to fat folks.

AJ: Oh, girl, you hit the nail on the head. I've been told I am 'a great candidate' for bariatric surgery, and at the same time I am told I am not healthy enough to withstand gallbladder surgery, which is medically necessary. Am I healthy enough to go under or not? Or is it just worth the risk if it will make me thinner? Not healthier, but thinner?

Nicola: Not well enough to have the surgery to fix what is 'wrong' with me (gallbladder), but well enough to fix my fatness.

AJ: And how much does a gallbladder weigh? Like, once I have that out will my BMI drop a bit? It's got to be *chunky* right now because it is *working* its ass off currently.

Nicola: It's wild! I found the only study that looks at anaesthesia risk with high BMI in IVF, and guess what it showed? Nothing. Class 4 folks, or however they classified it, did show a slight increase in mild complications, and that is it. When I looked further into it and was trying to find out what really impacts complication rates for folks going through egg retrieval it was things like surgery time and surgeon competency. Fat folks don't get access to the care, surgeons don't get the experience of operating on fat bodies: surgery was made and taught on thin people.

AJ: And they already have the implicit bias in them that it is riskier – this person is high risk because they are fat.

Nicola: We aren't born thinking that fat bodies are 'less than'. We don't look at trees and say this thin-shaped tree is better than this big, wide tree – we say both trees are trees, and they aren't better because of their shape. Wouldn't it be amazing if we stopped judging folks on their size or bodies like we do with trees?

We are born worthy. We are inherently worthy of every bit of care, support, tests, treatment or love that people need to grow their families. I wish that people knew that and could really embody that. Your body is capable of phenomenal things. Every day there are a billion things your body does that you have no control over; it does these incredible things, unconsciously. If we could sit there and appreciate everything our bodies do for us, that we don't have to sit there and think about making it move in a certain way but how it keeps us alive, how it keeps us safe. We are given this messaging of our bodies betraying us and not working as they should. Your body is on your team, it is trying to keep you safe, and it is trying to keep you alive. It is not working against you; it is doing its best to work against the culture and society that is telling you that you need to be smaller. Just knowing that your body is on your team, and you are working towards the same goal, can be incredibly powerful.

AJ: We are taught to battle our fat bodies, right?

Nicola: Yes! The idea of the thin person inside you that wants to get out – bullshit. This is me, this is all of me. It's scary to folks who benefit from the oppression of fat folks because if fat people are just as worthy, then where does their inherent worth now come from?

AJ: Last question then...what's your favourite fat people consumable? Like maternity bras, clothes or the like?

Nicola: My current favourite thing is my Snag leggings.

AJ: [gasp] They have pockets!

Nicola: They have pockets! Also, Big Sister Swap Shop. It's a company where you send the clothes that don't fit or that you don't like anymore. You fill out these surveys about your style and what you like, your size etc., and they swap out your bundle for things in your size and style. I also love Molke. I love their crop top-style bras too. I don't do underwired bras, especially after the pandemic.

AJ: The pandemic was the end of underwired bras for so many people!

Nicola: And jeans! I haven't worn jeans or an underwired bra since then!

AJ: What about maternity pants, or anything like that?

Nicola: I couldn't find them in my size, so I just got basic ones and washed them the best I could. One 'hack' that worked well for me was buying spaghetti-strap tops or tank tops and wearing them under my tops. I think it's called the one up, one down method. The tank top or spaghetti-strap top was under my top layer, so I could lift the top and my belly would be covered by the tank top, and then I wasn't having to worry about buying plus size feeding tops because everything was a feeding top now – I could just lift it up.

AJ: This is such a lifesaver because everything is now feeding clothes – lift it up and out of the way to feed.

Nicola: Especially because fat folks and clothing are so restricted; Yes, once I find something that makes me feel good, is comfortable and fits me, I'm not going to undertake the huge task of finding plus size clothing that is already a niche. And adding to that maternity clothing in plus sizes – forget that. I'll just wear what I have.

CHAPTER 4

Fat, Black, Queer and considering conceiving

Interview with Caprice Fox

Having interviewed Caprice for my first book, *Supporting Queer Birth*, I knew that I would want to speak with her again about her experiences of conception, pregnancy, birth and the perinatal period, with the lens shifting towards her experiences based on fatness.

Interview with Caprice Fox

AJ: I know we've worked together previously, but for folks who may be meeting you for the first time, how would you introduce yourself?

Caprice: I would introduce myself as a Black, queer woman. I use she/her pronouns. I am a primary school teacher and a freelance writer. I guess the relevant intro for this book would also be about my motherhood. My wife and I have one child, H. We are considering our options and starting discussions about having a second child. However, my apprehension, based on what I see online from other people in the same situation, as well as what I experienced in my first pregnancy, means that now, my BMI seems to be a big barrier to accessing conception and pregnancy services.

AJ: I guess, first and foremost then, before we continue discussions, would be for me to ask how to name or label yourself regarding your body. Do you use 'plus size', 'fat', or something else to describe yourself?

Caprice: I guess if it was in a formal setting I would use 'plus size' or 'curvy', but with conversations with my daughter, I am trying to own the word 'fat'. She's four and she is exploring and journeying with bodies. She will touch us and squeeze us, you know, my fat. She will say, 'Your stomach is fat' and I will say, 'Yes, my body has fat', just to explain it in a neutral and factual way – 'that's how our bodies store energy' – to try to ensure that there are no preconceptions about that word or the fat itself. Because, already at four she will have heard stuff and soaked in negativity surrounding fat. We are really trying to take ownership of that word right now.

AJ: It can take a lot of personal work doing that though, right? Because even when my youngest was small she would jiggle my belly and notice that my body was soft and warm and jigglier than most people's. And then force us really to unlearn these negative associations with our bodies because they are small and revelling in it. I would say things like you, like, 'Yes, it's so lovely and warm, soft, and jiggly, isn't it? It's lovely!'

Caprice: Yes, so when H says, 'Is your tummy fat?', I'll say, 'Yes it is', with a smile. This is just my body, and my body is home for her, it was her home, and it is close to me and my body that she feels safe. I don't want it to be a negative or a positive word, really, just a neutral descriptor of my body, and that is, that it is fat.

AJ: Yes, fat neutrality.

Caprice: We do touch on subjects like this at school, and I will have discussions with the children in my charge about these kinds of words, words that have historically been used loaded with negativity or used as a slur, for example. And that reclamation of language is about a community owning and reclaiming those words. 'Gay', in the past, has been used in school playgrounds as a negative. But me describing myself as a Black, gay or queer, fat woman...these are words that just describe me. It is just who I am and what I look like.

AJ: I also think it's about who is using those words, sometimes, for me. If I know someone who is also queer and they use the word 'queer' to describe themselves or someone else in the community, then that's okay. But if, for example, a straight-sized person named someone 'fat', it would make my ears prick up because of the history of hearing those words from straight-sized folks. In a similar way, if I heard cis-het (cisgender and heterosexual) folks using 'queer', I might, perhaps unnecessarily, fear that these are instances of reclamation of language, that these are being used in their negative, historical sense.

Caprice: Exactly, so when a new colleague at work asked me today if I had any plans for the evening and I said, 'Yes, I've got an interesting evening planned, I am speaking to an author about their new book! I spoke to them when they did their last book about queer birth', she looked at me like I had just said the most offensive thing in the world.

AJ: [laughing] That may or may not be why it's called *Supporting QUEER Birth* actually! Also, it's a huge reason why this book is called *Supporting FAT Birth* and not *Supporting LGBTQ+ Birth* or *Supporting PLUS SIZE Birth*!

Caprice: You know it's cool, babe, it's alright; some people use these words that you have, understandably, given the messaging of our world and media, assumed are negative, derogatory and otherwise nasty.

AJ: So for you, using these reclaimed words is neutrality.

Caprice: Yes. Fat, queer, Black are all neutral ways to describe myself.

AJ: You and your wife are approaching the possibility of a new conception, pregnancy and birth journey. With everything you said previously about what you are hearing and seeing about the treatment of fat folks in conception and pregnancy services, tell me more about that.

Caprice: When we first started trying, when we got married in 2016, we both put a huge amount of pressure on ourselves, as a lot of people do, to transform ourselves before getting married. That was what the service with the personal trainer was called, transformation services. I mean, I was completely transformed into someone who looked nothing like me. Looking back at the photos now, and although, of course, everyone has the right to look the way they want to look, for me, in those pictures... I was just so skinny; I didn't look like me. I didn't feel like me. My friends have since said that I wasn't, in terms of personality, like myself either. I mean, I was grumpy all the time. Tired, drained, hungry and lethargic. My fuse was so short too, quick to anger. I have also known, coming from my dad's side of the family, who are all Caribbean, and on my mum's side, from New Delhi and Staffordshire, that all the women in my family are curvaceous! That is just always how my body was meant to be and how it will always be. After the wedding we thought about trying to get pregnant, and everyone would tell us, 'You have to be in the best shape possible to be able to conceive', 'You need to be really fighting fit!' and they were telling me to lose weight, even though I had lost a considerably large amount of weight already. Looking back, I don't think it was the healthiest thing we did.

We went to a clinic, and they didn't weigh us; they didn't even ask us our weight. We got our first round of IUI (intrauterine insemination), and we got pregnant, first time. Which was great, but then, around four months into the pregnancy I was quite unwell. I had a very difficult pregnancy. From around four months pregnant I was using a wheelchair. My mental health was really suffering, and I was induced around 36 weeks or so. I had gone from being an active person to being signed off work from when I was four months pregnant, and obviously my mobility was vastly reduced. My wife was out at work most of the day and I felt trapped. It was soul destroying to feel so stuck. My mental health declined further and further with the isolation and lack of mobility; I was eating whatever was around me. I couldn't cook, I couldn't travel far to get fresh food and was relying on food that, I suppose, wouldn't be categorized as healthy. I, understandably, put on a lot of weight during pregnancy.

When I would go to midwife appointments, they started weighing me before I went into the appointment. And I saw that not everyone was being weighed. I had a bit of a dig around online and found out that I didn't have to be weighed. I could decline to be weighed at these appointments. I am still quite shocked, looking back now, that I had the courage to tell them I didn't want to be weighed anymore. I didn't necessarily go into too much detail about how it made me feel and what it was doing for my self-esteem and my mental health, because it was a huge, huge trigger for me, as someone who was bulimic for about seven years, throughout my late teens, university and just into my post-university life. I felt so listened to, they didn't weigh me anymore and I had weekly appointments and I was having quite a lot of appointments with my various complications, so they clearly did listen and take on board that being weighed was having a negative effect on my health.

Post-birth, it must have been six hours or so after giving birth, I was told...'You look so great, really, the weight is falling off of you already!' Those comments just carried on for a few weeks, and I know that when you've had a baby your body does change, and those are some of the factors people were commenting on, the puffiness depleting and my body rearranging itself.

Motherhood is something that I feel I was born to do. There aren't a lot of things that I will say with my entire chest, 'I am fucking good at this', but I know that I am a good mum, and I am a good parent. I think that I did neglect myself slightly; I don't weigh myself or look at numbers, but I do know that I have put on a lot of weight since I was pregnant.

Looking forward to today, I do know that there are restrictions about referrals to conception services based on BMI. Because we have always said that we would want H to be in school before we had any more children, people are now starting to ask us if we are going to start trying. I have seen recently four people who I am friends with or follow online who are having real issues even getting through the door of a clinic based on their BMI alone. They are weighed on the first meeting or the first consultation, and are told they need to bring their BMI down to under 29; for others it's 35 and some are 32. It is so frustrating to not know 'what is the line?' Because if it is a health reason, then fine, but if clinics are using a variety of 'cut-offs', then it can't be that folks in these numbers are unhealthy and folks in these numbers are healthy?

I know for them it is a numbers game and they have limited amounts of funding etc., but fat people can have babies. Fat people can get pregnant. It often feels like false concern, concern about health when it's a fatphobic issue and a funding issue, with them all having differing numbers and different criteria, and people are putting their lives at risk by frantically trying to lose weight in the fastest way to meet their criteria for funding. Being told you need to cut your BMI by 5 points in a matter of weeks before your appointment doesn't leave anyone with a healthy way of accessing those services. People will do it. I did, and I know other people who have done it because it is lauded as the only way to have your babies. It's just not okay; it is something that is a real worry for me. I don't want to have to be weighed when trying to access conception services a second time. We want to use the same clinic because we still have two vials of sperm, and we want the children to be full siblings. Plus, we've already paid for the sperm we have. We would be held hostage by their BMI cut-off in this situation. So, we must either abide by their restrictions, or not have access to our sperm and the choices we have made for how we want our family to be created.

AJ: Is the crash dieting something that you may have to consider, then? To access this clinic and your sperm? Which would mean an otherwise healthy woman, who has previously been pregnant and birthed a baby, with no underlying health conditions or concerns, at their current BMI is considering something that is known to be terrible for health

– crash dieting to meet the criteria so you and your wife can continue to grow your family in the manner that you have chosen.

Caprice: It would be the mental health side of things as well for me. My health, well, we know that wouldn't be great to put my body through this again, but emotionally, what it would do to me... I don't think... I, I don't think I could. I also want to consider what example I would be setting for H. For her to see me dieting. I don't want her to see me making her and my wife lovely, wholesome food and then I sneak away to drink cabbage water and hot peppers. It's not good for her. It's vile. But we are so limited. If push came to shove, I suppose, I would...I would have to do it.

Although when I lost weight for the wedding, I couldn't track my period. Since pregnancy and now that I am heavier, it is like clockwork. So that would also be a consideration with conception services being delayed or restricted while I am losing weight because I know the effect it has on my body when I am losing weight.

AJ: I know you are a breastfeeding peer supporter as well, and although I am going to talk more in-depth about lactation support for fat folks later, I couldn't pass up the opportunity to ask you what thoughts, if any, you have in this area.

Caprice: Well, I did my training when H was about four months. And we had what I would call a very easy journey. H fed well, she did the things she was meant to do, and between us, we had a very enjoyable and easy journey, we worked great as a team. However, there were instances where I was being given help or advice on positioning and they would want H down my body further and I would say, 'But my belly is there...how can I?'

AJ: A lot of the imagery in breastfeeding and chest-feeding in books, pamphlets and online resources shows skinny, predominately white women as well, perfectly spherical breasts with small, centralized nipples. Then once we add underarm fat, side fat, belly fat and the other variables of our bodies like nipple direction and size, the positioning and attachment of baby may need to look very different for fat folks than it does or might look for straight-sized folks. Our nipples' position and direction of travel may mean that generalized advice or information of tummy to mummy, looking up at the breast, neck and shoulders in line and tucked into your bod, won't work because, as you say...my belly is there! I think it's a wider symptom of the society we live in. I had never seen a baby being breastfed before I had my babies, and what precious little imagery or other exposure we do have to seeing someone nurse their baby is then almost exclusively white, cisgender, non-disabled, straight-sized folks.

Caprice: This is exactly the reason I am involved with setting up a new baby group, with the charity called Black Mothers Matter, to ensure that there are resources and support networks out there that have lived experience of accessing these services. It is a space for Black and mixed mothers and parents to gather in community and share resources, and it's so needed.

AJ: You can't be what you can't see, right?

Caprice: Absolutely.

AJ: Thinking forward slightly from the conversation we've had already about conception services, what about once you are pregnant and are moving through these services – what was your experience?

Caprice: My choices were very restricted in terms of birth plans etc. We felt as if we had done everything we could do in terms of getting ready for labour and our perinatal period... Holly gave me a massage every night to get my oxytocin flowing and she cared for my body and emotional wellbeing. I did hypnobirthing, we did the classes – we were ready to 'namaste' the shit outta this birth. I felt ready! But then it went downhill fast once I was using a wheelchair. I am, of course, not saying that I know how it feels to be a full-time wheelchair user or a disabled person. Additionally, my dad is a quadriplegic and a full-time wheelchair user. I remember speaking with him and he was very positive and encouraging about what the chair would unlock for me in terms of getting out and about, and how it is a tool for mobility. Very quickly, though, it was evident that it wasn't seen like that from the healthcare professionals' viewpoint. I felt very much that they had started treating me like I was stupid. The conversations would come from the assumption that I hadn't researched birth, I wasn't informed about anything at all, really, and I wasn't capable of advocating for myself. A lot of conversations started to be directed at Holly, and I would get frustrated at feeling ignored and would frequently speak up and say, 'I am here you know, I am right here!' I guess it amounts to a 'taster' of what disabled folks experience.

Our plan very quickly went from using the local birthing, mid-wife-led unit, which really appealed to us for lots of reasons, but primarily because it's small – there are just eight rooms, and it felt like the right place for us. However, they were now saying that I needed to be 'physically able' to be able to use the birthing centre, and it was no longer an option for us. They specified that I would have to independently be able to get on and off a bed, get out of a chair by myself etc., and the assumption that because I was using a wheelchair I couldn't self-transfer was immediate. I remember thinking, 'Wow, you have just restricted choice for a whole group of people'. We ended up at the local large university hospital; they took me down to theatre, like a theatre prep room, and I think I ended up giving birth in there. I can't quite remember.

AJ: Was the restriction to use the birthing centre purely based on your being a wheelchair user at that point, or was it your BMI too?

Caprice: I do know they have restrictions based on BMI, but I don't remember them ever bringing it up; it was just focused on what they perceived to be my lack of mobility. But when they place restrictions on BMI, particularly for Black and Brown women and people, it is biased. BMI doesn't consider Black and Brown folks, it doesn't consider muscle or breast weight; it's purely your height and weight. It was exclusively based on white, cis, non-disabled men. It is so outdated.

AJ: And it was never designed to be an indicator of health either! I mean, if I was a bit shorter, I am sure that I would experience fatphobia at an even greater level. Being 5 foot 10 inches, I think that helps me 'pass' in some instances.

Caprice: I remember having a similar conversation with Holly, actually. When we were working out and losing all that weight for the wedding, Holly wanted to work out her BMI. Holly has always been slim and slight all her life. But the 'body transformation' thing we were doing for the wedding just had her ripped! She was like Arnie! She could do one-arm pull-ups! So then we did her BMI and it was overweight! She had so much muscle and she looked like a body builder; no, she looked like Zena!

AJ: The ears of lots of queer folk reading this book have pricked up now at the mention of Zena, warrior princess, eh? Loads of memories as tweeny queers wondering why this TV show made us feel like our heartbeat was in our pants!

Caprice: Relatable! Very relatable! So Holly's BMI was high because of the muscle she had built.

AJ: It's interesting to consider the ramifications that categorizing people using such restrictive means like BMI will mean that folks like Holly, who are slight by their nature and healthy, could then be told that their BMI is too high. Possibly then they might be obligated to bring it down to access treatments or birth centres etc.

Similarly, when my dad was weighed, they would say that his BMI was just into the 'normal' category so that he was fine and healthy. But my dad was an amputee. There was no way of factoring in an adult male, minus a leg, in terms of BMI. I mean, he was 10 stone soaked through, and over 6 foot when standing; he was long and lean by nature, like Holly. They would still categorize his BMI based on equations that weren't accurate for him. Even though he is a white, European, cis male.

Caprice: It's just ridiculous. Using BMI to restrict or grant treatment when it is so inaccurate for so many people, for so many reasons; it's just heart breaking.

AJ: What should we be saying to the fat folk reading this book then? Given your lived experience, what do you want to say to them?

Caprice: Oh gosh, a lot. I think, primarily, education. Be as educated and informed as you can about your choices. A lot of things happen because we haven't said 'no' or objected. And yes, there are a lot of settings that have a policy and rules, but there are a lot that have phobic attitudes that are directing your care and treatment. There is no law or regulation against you declining their offer of a sweep, for example. Try to arm myself with as much knowledge as you can. That goes for all aspects, from conception to pregnancy and beyond. Having that knowledge is power. When folks say things like 'Fed is best' or 'Breast is best', it is simply 'Educated is best'. Informed is best, and knowing what is right for you and your situation is best. Also be ready to hear a lot of opinions from strangers and randoms about your health and the health of your baby based on your size. They will want to comment and touch you. You are allowed to stop them...

AJ: Oh, I backed up from plenty of offended folks in my pregnant past when they came at me with their hands out at belly height. Or said things like, 'Well, at least you're not showing, that's the benefit of already having a big belly, right?!'

Caprice: People will feel entitled to touch you and tell you that your body, baby or pregnancy can't be healthy because of your size.

AJ: I think it's so important for fat folks to hear this as well because it's

not just during pregnancy that we are told that our bodies are dangerous because of our mass. It is a wider societal problem, of course, that
birth is so often seen and portrayed in media as dangerous and always
an emergency, an inherently perilous situation. Further compound
those fears when your whole life you have been told that your body
is 'less than' – less healthy, less able, less brilliant – and abnormal...
We put fat folks at a disadvantage in empowerment of birth based on
fatphobia. Then, if that wasn't enough, fat folks are possibly going to
be told 'you have to' have a caesarean birth, 'you have to' be induced
based on BMI, 'you must xyz or you cannot xyz'.

I think it's a very pertinent point that you make that knowledge is
power in these circumstances. Not knowledge in the sense of committing to memory all the statistics surrounding interventions in birth,
but committing to our souls that we are 'in charge' here.

Caprice: Definitely, and I think that, for me, I feel a lot more in control
and informed going into this journey for a second time. I might have
already picked my doula before we've picked our clinic!

AJ: What about to HCPs then, what would you say to them?

Caprice: Being fat is not an illness. It is not a sickness, and fat people
give birth all over the world every single day. Fat people need and
deserve to be treated with respect.

AJ: I think so many people will think that is oversimplified, but it's
right on. It is a common lived experience of fat folks, in various
healthcare settings – that lack of respect. That lack of respect or
doubting our knowledge, autonomy or abilities.

Caprice: That is how I felt and how I was treated in pregnancy. One
of the best things was having Holly with me. She would always say,
'You know, we can take our time and think about it. We can go home
and have a discussion and take our time considering our options.' That
would be another nugget of advice from our lived experience I would

want people to know too: 'It is your birth; you can take your time to consider the options being given to you.'

AJ: Another question I am going to ask everyone is for their recommendations of where to go for maternity clothes and other-sized parenting paraphernalia.

Caprice: Bras! The best bras I found were from Elomi – they do nursing bras and underwear. They describe it as for the 'fuller figure'. They do bras up to a 48KK and swimwear up to a size 28. It's obviously not perfect, but they do go a lot higher than most high street places.

I also think it's worth pointing out that you can just wear 'regular' clothes and size up! I remember looking at maternity socks and thinking, 'Yeah, alright, I've got to have socks, so I'll need maternity ones!' It's clearly marketing a lot of the time, as I can just wear a floaty empire-line dress and size up a bit.

It's also important for me to pass on to other Black, fat, pregnant women and people to look at your elders, look at your families. See what the women in your family look like, what our bodies look like. It can be so far removed from the whitewashed imagery that we see surrounding pregnancy and motherhood. Seek out those safe spaces where you can be you.

Oh, and eat the Puff-Puff! Enjoy your jollof rice! Don't not eat the chicken! Eat the foods we've always eaten, for your body, and for your soul!

CHAPTER 5

Fat Birth

Interview with Dr Mari Greenfield

I have known and have worked with Dr Mari Greenfield for several years on many projects including my first book supporting queer birth and other birth world adjacent projects. Mari (she/they) is a researcher at King's College London, doula, birth and foster mum, and host of one of my favourite queer birth podcasts, 'Pride in Birth'. She is also a member of the Big Birthas team, so I knew I had to speak with her again for this book.

Taking advantage of their wealth of knowledge in so many areas of birth, I thought it might be best to ask a few burning questions I had, but to largely allow the conversation to flow and see where discussions surrounding fat birth led us!

I asked Mari if they would talk with me about what the research data says, and about their own lived experience of fat birth.

Interview with Dr Mari Greenfield

Mari: One of the themes of the research I carried out was when we were interviewing women who have had at least two children. We were talking to them about their first experience, which generally involved a lot of coercion. There was a theme that emerged where many of them felt that there was nothing that they could do to succeed (in their pregnancies). The NHS advice is that you should not diet while you are pregnant. We know that dieting during pregnancy is harmful. So they couldn't win. They couldn't lose weight without risk, but there is no way to win now – they are already a fat, pregnant person. The feeling was that the NHS wanted them to be very sorry that they got pregnant as a fat person, therefore apologetic the whole time that their body was bigger. And to agree with everything that everybody said: 'Of course I agree I can't have a water birth because my body is too big for you to manually handle me, even though my mass as a 5-foot woman with a BMI of 32 is less than a 6-foot person with a BMI of 29.'

AJ: Right? So I think one of the things I was not prepared for when I was a baby (new) doula was how strong people looked and how strong people are in labour. The perception is weakness and fragility, right? And, of course, labouring women and other labouring people are vulnerable and deserve safety, but they are far from weak and fragile. The manual handling concern is a common one. A lot of people are told you can't labour at home or in hospital in the water because they can't get them out quickly in an emergency. When Adam was asked, 'How will you get AJ out of the pool, quickly, in an emergency?' he said, 'I'll just cut it, it's a blow up, I will cut the pool.' The objection was, 'Oh, but your floors!' and Adam said, 'Well, if you are saying that it is such an emergency that we cannot wait for the contraction to finish or we can't give AJ a moment to collect themselves to help the four other adult humans in the room get them out the pool, then I'll cut it, fuck the floor.'

Mari: I looked and looked for data or instances of someone having to cut the pool to get them out in an emergency, and I've never found it.

AJ: I have had to cut one as a doula but not during labour – just where it got a slow puncture and we disposed of it afterwards.

Mari: But not in labour.

AJ: Oh no, this was afterwards.

Mari: I have heard all sorts, like 'Your home insurance won't cover any damage done by your birth pool', and all these other incredibly specific objections to home birth or water birth, and I couldn't find any documented instances.

In the piece of research I did that we were talking about before, with Big Birthas and parents who had a BMI of more than 30 in at least one of their pregnancies, they expected, in their first pregnancy, to be given evidence-based care. They expected that they would be given accurate, relevant information, and that they would make the decisions about their pregnancies and birth. They also expected that their BMI would be part of their discussions with their care provider, along with everything else that needed to be discussed. What they found was that once they had been labelled as 'high BMI' it over-shadowed everything else about their care. There was one interesting woman's experience whose BMI was under 30 in her first pregnancy and over 30 in her second. The difference in her weight was 7lbs. She had a completely straightforward pregnancy and birth at a birthing centre. She said that at every single appointment she felt scrutinized and criticized, and told her baby was going to die because she was too fat – all because of 7lbs difference. Other respondents said that every appointment damaged their mental health because they were told constantly that their baby's life was at risk because of their body size. There was also a theme on the assumption that a respondent's mobility would be impaired because of their BMI. What was done to 'help' with that was that women were given inductions and early epidurals and were therefore immobilized. So therefore they may not have had a mobility restriction, but they do now, because of the interventions offered.

Generally, people said, about their first pregnancies, that there was a lack of evidence-based care, a lack of respect, and they were hugely stressful. They also weren't likely to find out that they had the choice in the pregnancy and labour care until after their first labour. Some felt that they were deliberately misled in their first pregnancies, that they did not have the autonomy or right to choose their care for pregnancy or labour. Induction was one area that was mentioned in the lack of choice discussions. There are more experiences within this data set, like a woman who was told by her obstetrician that her baby was 'so big, he'll come out wearing school uniform'. She was, understandably then, so worried that she would tear during labour that she asked for a caesarean section, and the obstetrician declined this as there was no clinical need and she was left terrified because of this thoughtless 'joke'. Her baby was 7lbs 10oz. Another respondent was told 'you must have known that it was risky to get pregnant at your size', without checking if this was a planned pregnancy first. In this instance this was a pregnancy as a result of sexual abuse.

AJ: That is fucking horrific!

Mari: Isn't it just! Lots of the women after their first births had developed mental health conditions, which they attributed, themselves, in part as a result of the care that they had received. So next time round they wanted to make more of the decisions (surrounding their care), but they were faced with HCPs who were treating them exactly the same. All their efforts at negotiation, trying to practise informed consent and trying to decline scans and the like, they found were met with even more obstacles. Like being told that you cannot decline a scan, which, of course, you can. They were often told that not only by the obstetrician or the midwife but also by the admin staff who, when they called up to cancel their automatic invitation to a growth scan or an induction, would tell them, 'You aren't allowed to cancel' etc. This is just further evidence that everyone who works in a healthcare setting needs to understand informed consent. Faced with these barriers, some people just declined care. Some of that care was care that they wanted; they may have wanted to see an obstetrician to discuss something that wasn't about their BMI – for example, tearing or PPH [postpartum haemorrhage] in previous births – but they knew that the second they walked into an environment such as an obstetrician appointment at a midwifery clinic, that all they would discuss would be their BMI. There were also respondents who declined scans. There was one woman who had a possible partial placenta covering the cervix in her first birth; she thought that might explain why she had bled towards the end of labour and had had quite a high blood loss. She said she would have quite liked to have a scan in her second pregnancy to check the location of her placenta, but she knew that consenting to a scan would also mean foetal measurement being taken, which she didn't want. And then to access the results of where the placenta was, she would have to have an appointment with an obstetrician, which again, she didn't want. What this means is that women and other birthing people are not able to access antenatal services equitably.

AJ: This is interesting because on forums like Big Birthas I see quite often people saying, 'I wasn't allowed to cancel the appointment, so I am going to go but then I'll decline their offers of intervention when I am there.' I think your research and the lived experience of the women involved shows why there might be people who reply to that post with warnings of 'Be careful, because once you are in, and when that shift of patient/care provider happens of "I am in a gown now and here comes the people in charge in the white coats", it's harder to decline.'

Mari: That is definitely a factor, and there is another aspect to think about as well. If you are declining wanted care because you are scared, not having that care affects your mental health. People are also saying be careful because it is harder to decline care once you are in the healthcare setting, or they will be more reluctant to 'let you go' after you attend a setting, but people with lived experience know that even attending a setting like this can cause harm to pregnant people's mental health. Thinking about the woman who was told 'you must have known the risks before you got pregnant', that interaction has probably caused her trauma.

AJ: Almost undoubtedly, right?

Mari: If we want to look at the data about risk with pregnancy and obesity – if we even want to call it that – I don't particularly think it is the right word to be using. Because a set mass on one person can be considered obese, but the same mass on another person isn't obese, I don't think obesity is an accurate diagnosis.

AJ: Obesity is the medicalization of fat bodies, right?

Mari: Not even fat bodies, but heavy bodies...muscle weighs more than fat. There are people who are very muscley and who are classed as obese even though they have very low body fat. Particularly in kids, who are being classed as obese when they might be very muscley!

AJ: I had this thought the other day watching my youngest doing gymnastics and she was doing bar work and I could see her arm and back muscles and then she did a back bend, or a bow or something it's called, and I counted her eight abdominal muscles from across the room, super-strong!

Mari: Absolutely, my friend's son does BMX riding and his legs are about the same size as mine, but they are 100 per cent solid muscle, so when he was weighed at school, they were told he was obese. If we look at the correlates of people with a BMI of over 30 and what else in their lives goes with that, the number one thing is stress. So we are taking people who are already stressed and piling more stress on top with additional appointments and telling them their baby is going to die. The other biggest correlate for people with a BMI over 30 is childhood sexual abuse, in women. We are talking about taking people who are pregnant, already feeling down about themselves, and then compounding the stresses of living in a fat body and experiencing medical fatphobia and size bias, and this is a community or group of people where it's likely that a high percentage of them have experienced childhood sexual abuse. And then doing things to them and their vaginas with coerced consent.

AJ: And often with this air of 'It's your fault, you must have known the risks of getting pregnant' when it might not be a choice, and in 95 per cent of instances, like I discussed with Nicola Salmon, a person's mass isn't a variable that they can change. Which puts me in mind of one of the many phone conversations we've had about my gallbladder, where I was being 'prescribed' weight loss as a solution to my health difficulties. I wonder if there are any other treatments out there being offered with a 95 per cent failure rate.

Mari: Yep, nothing. The NHS insists that dieting works at the same time as reporting that more and more people 'have obesity' than ever before. This NHS treatment of 'prescribing' weight loss isn't new, so if it works, where are all the fat people coming from? We also don't have research about the long-term effects of being prescribed weight loss. We know that, generally, people are heavier after starting diets, regardless of the amount of weight loss initially, or how long they are in a 'maintain' phase; we know that in five years' time they are overwhelmingly likely to be just as heavy or heavier than when they started. What you then get is weight cycling and the risks that then poses to people's health, but where are the studies that confirm that is better for your health than just being fat? It would be interesting to look at things like the stillbirth rates of people who have had a high BMI consistently and have never tried dieting and compare them to people who weight cycle. We know that weight cycling is associated with people who have eating disorders; a common pathway there is people starve themselves and then binge eat because dieting is not a sustainable state, and can develop into bulimia. People are being 'prescribed' a treatment (weight loss) that isn't proven to improve out-comes; even on the rare occasions where a person is able to 'succeed' in weight loss, and actually, your mentioning weight, weight loss, weight management is actually likely to cause that person harm. Harm could be physiological harm in triggering an episode of eating disorders or other mental health-related conditions, or physical harm from weight cycling, including being overwhelmingly likely to end up weighing more than if you had said nothing.

AJ: There is also a discussion needed about the data and research groups within this too, right? Because if you treat everyone with a BMI under 30 the same and everyone with a BMI of over 30 the same, that doesn't give enough specific data about the risks or outcomes of those groups. There is too much variety within those groups, right? Like if someone's BMI goes over 30 for the first time and they have a BMI of 31 for 12 months after pregnancy, does that qualify them as 'over 30' in the same risk group as someone like me, who has been in a body with a BMI of 35–45 my entire adult life?

Mari: Yes, and if someone does a crash diet, for example, to get their BMI from 31 to 29.5 to get access to fertility treatment, they are likely going to end up heavier than when they started, when we know that fast weight gain during pregnancy is associated with a higher risk of stillbirth – much higher than having a high BMI to start with.

AJ: What would you change, Mari, if I gave you control now over fat birth in total, what would you change?

Mari: I think I would scrap BMI. I would not use BMI for any indication of health, or any indication of a person's mobility, or a person's likelihood of having this or that birth outcome.

AJ: One of my headings is 'BMI is bullshit', ha ha!

Mari: It so is. But if I had one thing to say to HCPs who are caring for pregnant people with a high BMI, although not necessarily just within maternity or perinatal services but all HCPs, is that the Hippocratic Oath of 'First do no harm' needs to be centred. A lot of the things that HCPs are doing are harmful, and the things they are saying have a high probability of being harmful for fat folks.

AJ: What would you like to say to fat pregnant people or for fat folks on a conception journey, or in their perinatal period, what would you say to them?

Mari: Choose the person or people who are going to be with you carefully. Consider taking someone with you to your scans, appointments or any interactions with HCPs. Choose that person carefully. Choose somebody who doesn't harbour fatphobia as well, and make sure that they understand their advocacy role. You are likely going to need an advocate to get through the NHS system without too much harm.

AJ: What do we say to the birth workers or the support people who are walking alongside the fat pregnant people? Are there any resources that you could recommend that they consume?

Mari: Most women who are overweight have a straightforward pregnancy and birth. Remember it is your job to advocate for them so they can be part of that majority.

AJ: Another question I am asking everyone is about their favourite consumable for fat folks, whatever that might be, fashion or the like, that you enjoy as a fat pregnant person or a fat parent.

Mari: If you have a bra already that fits and is comfortable, you can buy, from the internet, a clip that you can retro-fit to any bra to make it into a nursing bra.

AJ: Is there anything else that you want to say that we haven't covered?

Mari: Remember that this is *your* birth. If you find writing out a really highly detailed birth plan helpful, then do that. If you would find it more freeing to write nothing down, then do that... Don't let anyone tell you otherwise.

CHAPTER 6

Fat and Multipara

Speaking with Dr Mari Greenfield about the commonalities that many multipara (two or more pregnancies) mothers and other birthing parents experience got me thinking. My journey was very similar to what a lot of fat multipara mothers and other gestational parents choose to do second + time around. As Mari said in the previous chapter, their research found that a lot of second + time parents experience an intervention-heavy or a medicalized birth first time. Then, when they are pregnant for a second + time, they often opt for less intervention and a less medicalized birth. We also know that that second + time fat folks are even more likely to have a birth without intervention or an adverse maternal outcome than their first-time parent counterparts: 80 per cent of multipara parents with a BMI over 30.[1]

Thinking about these common experiences of wanting something different and usually markedly less intervention-heavy than the first time put me in mind of my pal Orla. I first met Orla when I was invited to Dublin to give an LGBTQ+ competency workshop to birth workers. Orla and I shared many similarities and histories, including being a fat person who had experienced fatphobia in our first pregnancy, which shaped our choices in our subsequent experiences.

Orla (she/her) is a breastfeeding counsellor who is pregnant for the third time. She lives in Ireland with her long-term partner in a blended family.

---

1   https://maternityaudit.org.uk/FilesUploaded/NMPA%20BMI%20Over%2030%20Report.
     pdf

Now for the fellow Irish folks and people with recent Irish ancestry, the following will make sense: I love Orla for many reasons, but handing me a Club Lemon and a bag of Tayto crisps in the bar of the hotel I was staying at in Dublin meant that the love was strong and immediate.

Interview with Orla Gallagher

AJ: I think the best place to start would be an overview of your journey so far, if that's alright? I imagine we are going to end up down some rabbit holes and chatting around the issues, so I reckon let's just start and see how we go!

Orla: Okay, cool. Although do tell me if I am going too far off-piste and rambling here! I was pregnant the first time when I was 17, and I was 18 when I gave birth. I have always been a Type A kind of person who reads the books, does the research, makes the lists and the plans. I like to know the terminology and be in control. I have always been that way. That is part of what can make pregnancy and birth so difficult, is that so much of it is out of your control, seemingly. I did a good amount of 'work' and I was aware of quite a lot, maybe not specifically to do with fat pregnancy and birth, but more about the general coercion that can happen. I went and sourced private antenatal education with an independent midwife. I do remember, though, that I was told by one of the social workers that they have a special class for teen mums and that I should be attending that. I had purposefully opted out of the hospital classes because, from what I had been told from other parents, those classes were to tell you about what policies the hospitals have. Not necessarily to inform you about the birthing process, or your rights as an expectant mum or parent; just to tell you 'This is how we do it here' kind of thing. So I did my birth plans. I had one that was my ideal world 'this is what I would want', but then I also made another plan for what if this happens, with another long list of stuff that 'I don't consent to' ahead of time, as well as a list of stuff that 'I do consent to' ahead of time along with further information about how I would like the interventions I do consent to carried out, and how consent should be sought regardless – I mentioned the Type A thing, right?

AJ: You don't need to now, babe, ha ha!

Orla: There were multiple plans! I brought my planner to an appointment that was quite late on, must have been 34, maybe 35 weeks. The consultant sat down with a biro and was crossing through things that wouldn't be possible, adding little addendums like 'Ideally I would prefer' in front of where I had written consent for 'intermittent monitoring', and then adding an asterisk to everything that said '*as long as everything is well with Mum and Baby*'. I wasn't thrilled but I just settled for the fact that there was engagement and discussion on my preferences. It didn't feel like I was telling them my boundaries and wishes; it felt more like a teacher going through my work with a red pen.

AJ: Not inspiring confidence, eh?

Orla: I was due in late November and there was, very unusually for Ireland, a snowstorm. We just don't get them here, too close to the water or whatever. I was at home and knew I was in early labour; I was getting surges and starting to feel uncomfortable. Over the Sunday it carried on like that, and then on the Monday morning, I knew the roads were quite bad, and so I thought let's head up to the maternity hospital because I was worried that if we left it any longer the roads might be impassable. When we got there the nurse was quite dismissive, saying, 'You aren't in labour, you've had an internal, we've put the monitors on' and all that craic. 'That's all we can do.' They never made it sound like going home was an option. She did say, 'You can go to the antenatal ward and hang about for a bit and see if things ramp up.' Knowing what I know now, I left my nice, cosy, safe, dark and comforting home, where I was starting to labour, then I got into the car, drove through this snowstorm to the big hospital with the bright lights and the alien environment, and everything stopped, or slowed to a crawl. I stayed in for a bit and they left me to do my thing, and I was surging and getting a bit of cramping here and there, but nothing major. By the Tuesday evening they said 'If you don't go into labour by tonight you will have to go home.' I was worried about the roads and going home and then labour ramping up again quickly and then the roads being even worse than before. They were also talking a lot, while we were in the antenatal ward, about how short-staffed they were – people couldn't get in because of the weather; they even said that the ambulances weren't getting back to the hospital – they were getting stuck on the roads etc. Going home sounded like a bit of a non-starter at this point. The next morning, I was still cramping and surging kind of off and on. The midwife came in and said, 'You aren't in labour, so we can either break your waters.' So I didn't feel that I had any other option but to have my waters broken. Had them broken, did the whole walk down to the hospital café walk around, and nothing was happening. They then said that because I had my waters broken that they expected me to deliver within 12 hours. I was progressing, I was walking about, labouring, doing my thing and progressing, but not to the timeline that they wanted. I think I was at 3cm for about three hours when they said that they would be starting me on a drip because I wasn't progressing. I knew that I didn't want to be on a drip because then I would be stuck on the bed with monitors on, and I didn't want that. I had been quite active the whole way through, walking around, finding comfortable positions to rest in for a while, and then having another wander about and finding another spot. I was also aware that when labours are augmented or induced, that it's harder to cope with the pain. When labours start and happen at their own pace, it builds up and your body better reacts and stuff. I was really worried that if they put the drip on, I wouldn't be able to move or cope with the pain. And that is what did happen. I ended up on the drip, and two hours later I broke.

I was in bits, after two days with no sleep. I was also in a two-bed room, two beds separated by a curtain in this slightly bigger than normal labour suite. I could hear everything the other person was saying to their partner, every grunt and every breath even. This was just not conducive to labouring at all. They did say, 'We will move one of you as soon as we can', and thankfully that was before either of us had our baby. Every time they would come in and talk to either of us about our labours, I was aware that if I could hear everything that she was saying or being told about her catheter or her piles, then she could hear me, too. I didn't really feel that I could move about freely or talk freely about what I wanted and what I needed. I also didn't think that I could ask questions or discuss my options properly because I was concerned I was disturbing her labours by talking or moving around. This was probably Wednesday afternoon, and I just knew it would happen. I saw it (interventions) happening, and it fucking did.

I was so cross with myself. I should have known better. I should have been able to better advocate for myself. I should have been able to foresee the cascade of interventions and all that craic. I carried a lot of guilt for a long time. Especially about getting an epidural because I was so tired, and I just couldn't cope with these sudden so intense and long contractions that the drip was causing. I had a really bad reaction to the drip, not only because I was used to moving my body and finding little spots where I was more comfortable, and now I was stuck on this bed, vomiting because I was reacting to this drip, being told to stop moving because the monitors weren't picking up baby's heartbeat.

Those monitors are just a 'dream' to have on you when you are fat – you know yourself, right? They kept getting cross that we couldn't get a good read and really shoving them into my stomach and making me feel like I was doing something wrong even though I was just lying there, existing. They then said about putting a 'little clip' on baby's head to do the monitoring instead. I didn't know it was more like a tiny screw into her head. When she came out, she had all these pin holes and marks all over her head from where they kept having to reattach it; I think it was five or six times they had to reapply it. Her head was in bits, I didn't know. No one actually told me it was going to be a little pin into my baby's head. I then felt awful about that as well, of course. I was on my back, epidural, coached to push, and it wasn't happening as quickly as they wanted, so again they said that they would make a little cut so 'we can help baby out'. That's how they said it. They didn't ask what I thought or if I would like to try a different position; they said, 'We are going to give you a little cut to help make more room for baby.' I was clear with them that my birth choices were clear – I did not want an episiotomy. I would rather tear naturally, if that was the case. But they said, 'Well, you've been pushing for ages, and you can't get baby out so it's either this or maybe forceps?' I thought, 'I don't want to go to theatre, I don't want forceps', so again, I had to go with their first offer of an episiotomy. I didn't really have time to make peace with it, but I was thinking, 'Okay, this is the price I have to pay to get my baby out.' Knowing what I know now, I might have done something differently because I was on my back, with an epidural, being coached to push, with no discussion about changing position at all.

AJ: That's a lot, are you okay? Do you need to stop? We can stop if you need to.

Orla: No, I am okay, the pregnancy hormones aren't helping though!

AJ: Just let me know if you need to stop, okay?

Orla: Thank you. At the time, I don't think I would have named any of it as traumatic or trauma. It wasn't until after and I was looking back or talking to other people about my experience. It was the fact that I had no agency. Even though I had done the work that I had done, sought out education, prepared myself in every way I knew how. I just still had no autonomy. I didn't feel like I was participating in what was happening; it was very much 'this is what we do here'.

AJ: Oh darling, I am so sorry that happened. You are not alone. It doesn't make it right, of course, but you are not alone. There are so many women and other birthing people who felt that birth was something that happened to them rather than something that they did.

Orla: It's the anger, too. At this stage, it's not that I am upset or crying about what happened to me; I am pissed, and I am crying because it is still happening. Every single day. Also, it could have been so different. The day I presented at the maternity ward, in early labour, if I had met a midwife who listened, and rather than saying, 'You aren't in labour', if she had said, 'You know, I hear you, something is happening, but sure, it's your first baby. You could be here a while. You might be more comfortable at home, would you not? We are here, come back whenever you need us, but go home, have a bath and a nap if you can. When you hit the 10/5/3 ratio, come back!' I was 40 + 1 with my first baby, so there was very little reason that I needed to stay in the ward that night. Everything was well with me and my baby; there wasn't a good reason to induce me, other than I was already in the hospital. Sure, the weather didn't help matters, but no one ever told me I might be better off going home. No one even told me I was allowed to go back home. Or that coming in could have stalled things or slowed them down. Being younger and bigger played a part in that treatment, I believe. While I am white, I was in my hometown, I had accessed antenatal education and I was sure of myself, this still happened to me. For sure, what you said about birth happening to me, the whole experience, back in 2010, really influenced me and made me so sure that I wouldn't be doing it *that* way again.

AJ: What was different, then, the second time round, and what, if anything, do you hope will be different the third time round?

Orla: I went in with just an absolute zero tolerance for anything other than the level of care that I would accept for myself. The way that I advocated for myself from the outset was hugely different. I wanted to sort out private midwifery care for a home birth, but we ended up unable to access private midwifery – between the distance away that the closest midwife lived, and the fact that it would cost us about

€6000. We had also moved, and it wasn't the same hospital as before; it was a birth unit in a large hospital rather than a standalone maternity unit. But as I said, I just went in with that zero tolerance.

AJ: What does that look like in practice? Can you give any examples?

Orla: For me it was things like saying to the GP when the referral to maternity services was being done, 'I do not want this consultant named on my referral' – who I knew was particularly fatphobic and intervention-heavy. I also showed up to my booking appointment and made it very clear that I was not going to be stepping on the scales. I told them that I wanted midwifery-led care and not consultant-led care. I didn't fit into the low-risk box because, guess what? I am fat.

AJ: [faux surprise] No? Ha ha!

Orla: So then my zero tolerance looked like asking for an individualized risk assessment of me not based on the general pathways; I wanted them to consider me as an individual. They didn't agree to do that, but they did say that they would 'see how things go'. I was pretty sure that they were convinced that I would test positive for GD [gestational diabetes] or some other complication that they could then use as 'proof' and get me off my soap box requesting midwifery-led care. I also told them that I wouldn't be getting weighed at any of my visits, and that I didn't want any discussions based solely on my BMI. I knew that BMI was a risk factor; I already knew exactly what they thought of me being fat; I didn't need it to be discussed at every visit. I didn't want their advice or opinion on my BMI. Because I am here, and I am fat already, so there is fuck all we can do about it now, lads. Telling me I am fat at every appointment isn't going to change that.

AJ: What was their reaction to that? Did they accept that?

Orla: The GP said, 'I can't send the re-referral without your weight. The system will reject it if I send it blank.' I said, 'Well, I will stand on the scales and you can make a note of the number, but I don't want to know, I don't want you to tell me or read out the number or write it on any other of the documents that I will see.' At this point I was properly about three years into HAES (health at every size), and having a 'fuck diet culture! Diets don't work' mentality. So I was pretty adamant that I would not accept this behaviour. The GP still read the numbers out the second I got up on the scales, of course.

AJ: For fuck's sake!

Orla: He also grabbed my leg at another appointment, squeezed it and said, 'Are you sure you aren't swollen?! Because you look really swollen.' Didn't ask to palpate me, didn't even warn me – just lent over and squeezed my leg.

AJ: Isn't he a brave man, all things considered?

Orla: I did whip my leg away rather fast and said, 'My legs are fat. I know how big my legs are. I am fine. Don't touch me without my consent again.' I did fire him, eventually, but at this point I was still just trying to get on to the system and get access to midwifery-led care. Then, when I did get to my booking appointment, the midwife said, 'Have you ever thought about losing weight?'

AJ: [literally up in arms] Never! Who are these HCPs who are asking fat women about weight loss as if we don't live in a society that tells us from our preschool years we need to be smaller? Who are these people?! 'Have you ever considered…' Jesus wept.

Orla: I lost it, I went on an absolute tirade. First I asked her to repeat herself. I said, 'Sorry, what did you say?' and she repeated it!

AJ: Auk! You gave her an out and everything!

Orla: She even said, 'Have you heard about Slimming World?! Some people say great things about Slimming World!'

AJ: To a pregnant woman! Slimming World!

Orla: I informed her that as a fat person who has been fat my entire fucking life, yes, I have considered losing weight. I have spent nearly my whole life on diets, from the age of ten, when I first went to WeightWatchers. This started a long history of disordered eating in my life. And you know what? They always make me heavier. They always fuck with my mental health, which then, in turn, fucks with my physical health because I can't take care of myself as I usually do. I had an older child in school already at this point as well, so I was at the forest school helping out running the sessions, I was up and down, walking the dog. I felt great; I was probably at the healthiest I had ever been. She didn't ask me about any of that, or what I eat or what I do all day. She just asked if I had considered losing weight. I told her to never ask somebody that again. That one question could be enough to fuck everything up for someone who was in recovery from an eating disorder or someone who experiences disordered eating. That could be the last nail in the coffin. Asking people who society tells should be looking in the mirror and wishing they were smaller and doing everything possible to get there, even to the detriment of their mental and physical health.

AJ: We know you are right, of course (see the COBWEBS model);[2] this is not only pointless because I am pregnant now and our own NHS tells us it's bad to lose weight in pregnancy, so it's pointless to recommend dieting to me right now, as it's more likely to cause harm than to have a positive impact on my health.

Orla: Oh, we went through that. I told her every time that I have intentionally tried to make my body smaller it gets bigger. I knew

---

2   https://pubmed.ncbi.nlm.nih.gov/24997407

I didn't have to justify myself, but I wanted her to understand the harm that she could do, the harm she likely has done. I know that based on the number on the scales they are going to consider me to be high risk, so 'Let's do the tests! Let's do the GTT [Glucose Tolerance Test], let's take my blood pressure, let's get a blood test sent off before you make a decision that will impact my choices during pregnancy and ultimately my birth based on the number on the scales alone. If your only concern, about mine or my baby's health, comes from the number on the scales, then I am not entertaining that. Let's confirm that there is a risk before we resign ourselves to a "high-risk" birth.' They wouldn't clear me to go on the midwifery-led pathway until I had a clear GTT because I hit the BMI risk factor. I thought fine, let's do it, because they said that if it was negative there was no reason that I couldn't have midwifery-led care. So I wasn't told an awful lot about the appointment, just that I would have bloods taken and that I shouldn't eat after midnight. I rocked up and immediately realized there had been a mistake because I was supposed to be fasting since 8pm! An 8am blood test and a 12-hour fast. They said, 'Let's carry on because we are here', and someone from the dietetics department rang me and said, 'I've had your details over; I need to book you in for your care from us.' Now I hadn't had a call to say what my results were, but I knew enough to know it's not a positive or negative situation. It's based on a range of blood glucose levels, right?

AJ: Yes, and those can vary across hospitals and time, of course.

Orla: Totally. So she said my fasting number was just over and the other two results were fine, which totally confused me as to how they got to a gestational diabetes diagnosis based on just one of the figures being slightly off. This obviously wasn't completely accurate because I hadn't been told to fast for 12 hours and the other bits and pieces about water and ensuring that you eat normally in the days leading up to the test and everything. I said that I wasn't happy to accept these results and asked if we could do it again. She wasn't sure herself and said that she would get someone to call me back.

Eventually, when the sister called me back and was quite confused about why I wasn't just accepting what I was being told, she said that she could book me in for another test. There was a moment where I thought, well hopefully it won't be worse than last time, but having been given the proper information I fasted for the correct amount of time and everything was fine, and the results were under the cut-off.

AJ: That is a lot of self-efficacy, knowledge and advocacy to get access to midwifery-led care! An awful lot.

Orla: It is, and it's only because I took that zero-tolerance line of 'I won't accept anything less than individualized care' that it happened.

AJ: So easy to see how so many people get swept up in conveyor belt care, isn't it?

Orla: Totally! I still had to see the obstetrician and their team at each hospital appointment at around 36 weeks, and one doctor tried the old 'We'll book you in for an induction', even though there were no concerns throughout the pregnancy with my health or baby's health, and everything was going well. I wasn't even at term yet and the doctor wanted to book my induction. I declined their offer and said that I would come back to them if I changed my mind or if any risk factors developed. But there was still that fight or 'no, no, this is what we do' expectation that I just wasn't fitting into.

AJ: Your stance of 'I am not accepting anything less than the care I want, need and deserve' – did that carry through into labour?

Orla: Yes, I was 40 + 3 due to go in that day for an antenatal. I woke up that morning a bit crampy and something was going on. But I wasn't convinced. I had done a 10km forest walk the day before, so I thought maybe I am just sore. I had also been up to Dublin there for my dad's 60th a couple of nights before, up singing with the band and the rest of the craic there. I had done my very similar birth preferences document that I had for the first time round. I had about 17 copies of that document with me; I could have given one to everyone I saw, even the porter who took us up – if he was after one, I would have had it. But I called them up and said, 'I am not a DNA (did not attend) for today, I am not coming on purpose because I think I might be in very early labour.' The midwife was great; she said, 'Auk sure, you know yourself, second baby, we're here if you need us' and all the rest of it, right?

AJ: Perfect! I love how it was kind of exactly what you wished they had said to you the first time round. Like, 'we hear you, we believe you, we're here when you need us', like.

Orla: Absolutely, and I just put the immersion on for a bath, had a cuppa and went back to my ball with some tunes on while I waited for the water to heat up. I texted my other half and said, 'No rush, like, but leave at lunchtime and come home.' He got called to an emergency on the way home, and so by the time he got back and had got showered after being in a factory all day, I was pretty sure that I wasn't going to be sent home not being in established labour anymore! Because, as I mentioned before, this was a maternity unit in a larger hospital – we had to park at one end and the maternity unit was right up the other end. You have to walk like a full kilometre to get to the birthing unit! I walked the first long corridor, no problem, but then, after it bends round and opens up to another long bit, I couldn't take more than a few steps without having to stop and wait for the contraction to pass. Every ten steps or so I had to stop and work through these contractions. It took a while for us to get up there, but by the time we were there I knew we were getting places now. I wasn't worried that I was going to have the baby in the corridor, but I knew things were moving on. So, by the time we got to the desk, and they usually want you to do the forms and get everything signed and ready to go before you go onto the ward or into the birthing suite, right? The midwife looked at me, waited for that contraction and said, 'Ah sure enough, we'll do those later, shall we? Let's go in here so', and gently guided me into a private room. I gave her a copy of my birth plan and she said she had already looked it up when I called in and she had seen it, but 'I'll take another copy', she said, 'to make sure it's out in the room for anyone else to have a look at too.' Then she offered to get the shower running if I wanted some water or, 'Do you want to try the ball? I can get one of those down for you if you like.' I remember just thinking, 'Gosh, this is just so different, and you are just saying the right things!'

AJ: 'Where the fuck have you been?' Ha ha!

Orla: Ha ha, absolutely! She just immediately believed me and started suggesting things that fit my birth plan and my preference sheet rather than telling me what I could or couldn't do. She read and respected my choices in my birth plan and offered tailored options for me. She said, 'I know you don't want to have the continuous trace on, but can I get a base line reading while you are comfy here on the ball?' Then when I wasn't comfy on the ball anymore, she asked me how I had been coping at home – did I find any position that was more comfortable than others? I said I had been leaning on the kitchen counter and I found that worked well!

AJ: The amount of people I know who labour against kitchen counters or kitchen tables! That 'bent at the waist and supported on the forearms with the swaying hips'. That's the one. That's how I laboured with Emma. Next to my fridge, in fact!

Orla: Absolutely, so she cleared off the bed and got it raised up so I could lean over the side of the bed like the countertop at home! Then when I was comfy she said, 'Could I kneel down and get the Doppler on for a quick read?'! Again I was grand with this. After a little while I said to her, 'I might quite like to know where we are at, for my own peace of mind.' She said, 'Okay, did you want to ask me anything about that or how would you feel if it's not what you were thinking?' etc. She was fab. I said, 'Yeah, I hear you, but I want to have an internal to know where we are at.' I knew things were progressing and I knew it was all happening but I think, again, because of the lack of control aspect I thought having a number and knowing where I was at would help with that.

AJ: Fab.

Orla: She said I was around 8cm. I was ecstatic. I said, 'That's absolutely class, I have done so well, I am incredible etc. I have done all this by myself.' I was fucking made up. So then I felt like I could completely concentrate on labouring. Tom and I, we were just laughing through the contractions really, we have quite a typical Irish relationship where we show love through taking the piss, basically, and the midwife was joining in, we were gently ribbing each other and it was just so nice.

AJ: It sounds it!

Orla: It really was, and she was gently suggesting things like, 'How about the ball, would you be ready to try the ball now?' and, 'I can get the shower going if you want to try that?'! She had clearly read my birth plan and was using that to make active suggestions to try and help me through labour.

AJ: Day and night, then, compared to your first experience.

Orla: When I got to the point of transition [the last part of active labour] I was saying and thinking, 'I can't do this', 'I couldn't do this last time', and things like, 'Last time I couldn't cope and needed the epidural', so those thoughts were in the back of my mind. My midwife simply said, 'You are doing it, you have done it.' She reminded me of what I knew, but in that moment, just couldn't remember. It was perfect. She was even saying back my affirmations to me; one I loved was 'My surges can't be stronger than me, because they are me.' She ended up hovering underneath me, ready to catch baby as I stood, next to the bed, as I birthed my baby.

AJ: Birth workers do it in all positions after all!

Orla: Ha ha! She then passed baby up to me and she said, 'Don't bring her all the way up just yet', but I heard 'Bring her all the way up' and unfortunately the cord snapped. She was as cool as a cucumber and didn't make me panic at all. She just said, 'When you are ready, maybe get up on the bed and we can get you sorted.' But I could see my other half looking a bit worried and so I asked him, and he said, 'It's a blood bath!' I looked down and it was everywhere. It had sprayed all over the bed, the floor, the midwives, my other half, the walls – it was everywhere! The midwife was just so cool and calm, just really reassuring. When we got onto the bed and everything settled a bit she said, 'Although we're almost certain that this is cord blood, how would you feel about a managed third stage?' [giving medication to contract the uterus to assist in the delivery of the placenta], because they wanted to ensure that the placenta was whole and the blood wasn't from anywhere else. We had already talked about a managed third stage and I had told her how sick the Syntocinon had made me feel in my first labour, but she reassured me that they could use an alternative medication that hopefully wouldn't have the same effect. It really was a conversation about 'How would you feel? I know you didn't like it before, but there is an alternative. Do you have any questions?' It wasn't a healthcare professional saying 'you've got to' or 'you must' or 'you're not allowed'. She was telling me why and asking my thoughts.

AJ: Again, day and night!

Orla: It was, it really was. I felt absolutely fantastic the entire time. We were together skin to skin for about 90 minutes and I went and had a wee shower of my lower half and came back and got all snuggled up again with baby and just felt incredible.

AJ: What, if anything, Orla, would you say to fat folks about fat pregnancy and labour? You've had two very different experiences and are looking down the barrel of the third, so I wonder what information you would pass on?

Orla: Don't wait for anyone to give you permission. Take your autonomy and don't wait for a clinician or a healthcare professional to give it to you. You don't need them to agree with your choices; they are your choices. Say to yourself, out loud if you would find it helpful, 'I trust my body.' I trusted my body to give birth as I trust it to do the other countless functions it does daily. I don't question my body's ability to digest my food or remember to breathe, so why would I start questioning it now? Just because the system pathologizes fat pregnant people, well, pregnant people in general, but particularly fat pregnant people, doesn't mean that I cannot do this. That my body cannot do this. I was also, as I mentioned before, really up front with my healthcare professionals about what I would and wouldn't accept. I would have those uncomfortable conversations where I would say, 'I know you are working within a system that wants you to complete this form, tick this box and whatever, but I am an individual and this is the minimum that I will accept in my care.' Which I appreciate takes huge amounts of privilege to be able to do. I said, on more than one occasion, 'I am more than my BMI and I am not willing to allow that to dictate what my pregnancy should or shouldn't look like.' I also had to do a lot of work to unlearn my own fatphobia.

AJ: Is there a favourite fat parent product or consumable that you would recommend to other fat parents?

Orla: Yes! As a fat parent that used slings and carriers a lot, I really liked my Kinderpack carrier. Kinderpack has a 'plus size' strap option on their carriers. I haven't seen that on any other brand. I found other buckle and webbing-structured carriers really uncomfortable, but these have padding all the way to the end of the straps so it doesn't dig into my rolls. It's also a really small family company so it feels good supporting them over the larger factory manufacturers. Oh, and Birkenstocks! When you get to the point where you just can't bend down to lace your shoes, I can just stomp my feet into my Birks and I am away!

AJ: Birks or Docs for life. Hot: Birks, cold: Docs!

Orla: Sounds like a plan!

AJ: What would you say to the healthcare professionals or the birth workers about caring for fat pregnant people?

Orla: It sounds ridiculous, but treat us like people. We are just as worthy as any other service user. We see the looks or the slight recoil in your touch when you must palpate us – we know, we can tell. Do the work, unpick your fatphobia, work out why you think that way in the first place. Be open to acknowledging the impact that your fatphobia has on your practice. Sit with the discomfort of knowing that you've probably given people substandard care because of your internalized fatphobia. And your internalized misogyny, your racism, your homophobia, your transphobia – all that shit. We all have work to do to get to being anti-bias, whatever that bias is, we all have work to do to get there. We have to be willing to do the work and we have to be willing to admit we are wrong in order to do that.

CHAPTER 7

Pregnancy and Birth Choices

Navigating maternity and perinatal services can, understandably, feel like an alien world. All these new words, abbreviations and assumptions can leave your head spinning. On top of navigating the services, pregnant folks are often also trying to traverse work, parental leave, preparing physically and emotionally for baby, listening to everyone and anyone who feels that they can touch their bump, tell them all the birth or parenting horror stories they can think of, getting to grips with folding the buggy, envisioning their new world and the new person soon to be there with them. Fat folks are likely dealing with more frequent appointments, tests and referrals as well as the fatphobia and weight bias within their appointments.

I think right off the bat we must have a reminder. Straight out of *Am I Allowed? What Every Woman Should Know BEFORE She Gives Birth* (Beverley Ann Lawrence Beech, 2014, p.1.):

> A Government Report 'Changing Childbirth' (Department of Health, 1993) made it clear that the government expects the rights of women to be respected... Women must be the focus of maternity care. She should be able to feel that she is in control of what is happening to her and able to make decisions about her care. Based on her needs, having discussed matters fully with the professionals involved.

Your BMI doesn't supersede these rights. All treatments, tests, interventions and scans are offers. Even though seldom presented as offers, NICE (National Institute for Health and Care Excellence) confirms:

'A pregnant women is entitled to decline the offer of treatment such as caesarean section, even when the treatment would clearly benefit her or her baby's health. Refusal of treatment needs to be one of the woman's options.'[1]

One of the ways I found helpful to consider my options when offered an intervention in my pregnancies, and one that I share with anyone I brush up against who opens the topic, is the BRAIN acronym:

B: Benefits. What are the benefits of what is being offered? Example: 'It may be beneficial to have an epidural fitted in advance of established labour as you will be more comfortable and better able to remain as still as possible for the fitting of the epidural.'

R: Risks. What are the risks of the intervention being offered? Example: 'Can you tell me the risks of breaking my waters versus waiting for them to break spontaneously?' Note: No intervention is risk-free, and any assertion from HCPs that any augmentation or intervention is risk-free is to be addressed with polite, but firm, questioning.

A: Alternatives. What alternatives to your offer of treatment are available? Example: 'I am not sure about continuous monitoring as it will restrict my movement in labour; what are the alternatives?'

I: Intuition. What is your gut saying? This is often much easier said than done. It might be helpful to have this discussion with a loved one or your chosen support person. You are also allowed to ask for time to consider your options and to discuss their offer of intervention in private.

N: Nothing. What happens if we do nothing? How does that affect the benefits, risks and alternatives? Example: 'You've offered to fit intravenous Syntocinon to "speed up labour", but what happens if we do nothing and allow labour to naturally progress?'

---

1   www.nice.org.uk/guidance/qs132

You may go round these discussion points more than once, and you do, of course, always retain the option to change your mind, at any point.

You would be forgiven, especially if you have read *This Is Going to Hurt* (Adam Kay, 2018), for having the assumption that birth plans are exclusively for, as Kay put it, 'floaty-dressed mother(s)' with a 'nine-page birth plan, in full colour and laminated'.[2] A birth plan is for you if you feel you would find it useful.

It might also be useful to consider the purpose of the birth plan. Seldom is it a rigid, unmoving and uncompromising play-by-play that labouring people will never deviate from. The act of writing a birth plan isn't just to decide, forever more and come what may, what is going to happen when you have your baby. Considering your options, what is or isn't acceptable to you, given your past experiences and individualized needs, is the point.

Talk through your worries, as well as what excites you about your birth (this is allowed, contrary to the popular portrayal of labour and birth). In discussion, you may find what excites you, what might empower you.

You may have absolute non-negotiable boundaries such as no to vaginal examinations. You may be told that this is against hospital policy or against their guidelines. They are, however, *their* guidelines and not yours. You are entitled to decline any and all offers of examinations, investigations, scans or any other interventions. You may have some that you would hope to avoid unless necessary or there is an immediate risk of harm. Additionally, you may have something that you are happy for the HCPs in attendance to offer you. I had a list of things that HCPs could do without talking to me first. This included using a Doppler to listen to baby, take my blood pressure or my blood glucose level. I also requested that they didn't disrupt the silence to ask for permission to perform these tasks, and that they carried them out without turning on the big light (I provided torches, although most medics will have them).

Western society is doing its best to separate pregnant women and

2   www.aims.org.uk/journal/item/obstetric-violence-media

people from their autonomy, especially with the current political landscape that we all live under post *Roe v. Wade* in the USA, and even on this side of the Atlantic we had Baroness Nicholson tabling a now prorogued bill at the House of Lords, to lower the time limit for abortion to 12 weeks.[3] Despite the inane messages from the wider global north of society, you do not become solely an incubator for the unborn and lose your complete and utterly unshakable right to bodily autonomy. There are zero provisions, addendums or appendices to this most basic of human rights. Your fatness, Blackness, queerness, disability, age, class or status of any kind do not dissolve this most sacred of rights. Autonomy, autonomy, autonomy, always, always and forever, autonomy: 'Bodily autonomy is the foundation upon which all other human rights are built.'[4]

So, when considering, in your birth plan, whether you can indeed decline that intervention or not, remember: the right to decline an offer of treatment is what bodily autonomy and consent in medicine is built on. Without the very foundation of 'you can decline', then treatment cannot be consented to. Consenting to treatment because of lack of other options or due to coercion of medical professionals, or even loved ones, isn't consent; it is coercion.

---

3   https://bills.parliament.uk/bills/2028
4   www.unfpa.org/press/bodily-autonomy-fundamental-right

CHAPTER 8

Big Birthas

When the idea of this book was still kicking around my head, I knew that if I was going to write it, Amber Marshall (she/her) of Big Birthas would be the first person on my list of interviewees.

Amber, for anyone unaware of Big Birthas and the incredible community she has created for fat pregnant women and people, founded Big Birthas in 2011 with the aim of creating a supportive, evidence-based community for people who are, have been or would like to be pregnant with a higher BMI.

In Amber's intro blog she says, 'After an easy pregnancy and birth, I was initially astounded and then angry to discover it wasn't luck that I'd avoided all the complications presented as almost inevitable; it was always a likely outcome for someone with my BMI and no other health concerns.' She continues:

> while I experienced some excellent care in my second pregnancy, I faced an uphill battle from some professionals regarding home birth and was shocked at their tactics to browbeat or guilt me into submission; asserting vehemently (and incorrectly) that I wasn't allowed... They would sensationalize the true picture using relative risk statistics to claim my pregnancy was 'high risk', rather than marginally higher risk. I feel strongly that it's not fair, accurate or proportionate to care for people in this way. Or to restrict options without an evidence base, I felt this practice needed highlighting and challenging. Through the website and Facebook group, the community supports women and people to understand and contextualize the messages we're given in

order to make truly informed choices. We advocate for the respectful, appropriate, collaborative person-centred care we all deserve. I now serve on a number of committees and research groups as an 'expert by lived experience', helping to inform policy and ensure researchers are asking the right questions.'

I sat down with the woman herself, over Zoom, to chat all things Big Birthas and fat pregnancy.

Interview with Amber Marshall

AJ: Where do we start, Amber?

Amber: Well, I think in general, things are improving...but not by much. I have been in this field for the last nearly 12 years. Back then you had precious little chance of getting into a midwife unit. You were off to the obstetric unit. That was certainly my lived experience first time round. Second time I said I was having a home birth and I did, and it was fabulous. We are seeing more people getting into birthing units now and sometimes that is under the guise of wanting a home birth and then a compromise is made to allow access to the midwife-led unit instead.

AJ: Some people might not be aware of these situations, so, for clarity, this might look like someone being told that they can't access the midwife-led unit because of BMI and they then state they are having a home birth and the midwife-led unit may then be offered as a compromise. Sometimes that is a bit of a 'wink wink, nudge nudge' situation, where the service user might not actually want to have a home birth, but their provider might offer the birthing unit as a compromise, because they would rather have them in a healthcare setting than giving birth outside of a hospital entirely. Sometimes folks do want a home birth and they may still be cajoled into the birthing

---

1   www.bigbirthas.co.uk/about-big-birtha

unit under the basis of risk management and ease of intervention, should it be necessary.

Amber: Absolutely, also equally, however, we have seen situations, as was my lived experience, where people are then told, 'Yeah, you can use the midwife-led unit' and then they turn up on the day, in labour, you know, slightly preoccupied, to then be told, 'No, you cannot access the midwife unit because of your BMI' – which really destroys trust in our providers. There are, of course, entirely different experiences across the country where people are getting great care and having much more balanced conversations on risk. We see that in experiences being shared in Big Birthas where they have been told, 'Yeah, your BMI is a bit high, but without any other indicators of risk, go for it!' It is patchy. In some ways that makes it better, and in some it makes it worse. Sometimes it feels out of reach for folks in areas where there are much stricter cut-offs and much more emphasis put on BMI as the sole indicator of health.

AJ: Oh absolutely, and even from one pregnancy to another we see that difference in treatment. That was my experience certainly. When I went to my 30-odd-week appointment with the obstetrician when I was pregnant for the second time, with Emma, and told her that I was birthing at home, I was poised for push-back and a lot of fight in my choice, but she simply sat back in her chair, glanced at my notes, and said, effectively what you summarized before, 'Yeah, your BMI is higher than we would like, but in the absence of any other risk factors, go for it.' She did say, 'You are losing weight as well, which is great.' I mean, I weighed less at 30-odd weeks than I did at booking [appointment], which we know isn't great...

Amber: Ah yes, this is a common experience as well, if you are losing weight (at a hell of a rate, once you consider the increase in blood, amniotic fluid, weight of baby, weight of placenta and the rest of it)! Half the time it's still praised as 'good for you' to be losing weight.

AJ: It feels as if, at any point, and at any cost, it's great to weigh less because fat = bad, so less fat must be better. Although we know that most fat women and people have a normal pregnancy and birth we would be forgiven for assuming that there were whole vast oceans of proof that fat = bad and dangerous for parent and baby.

Amber: We can't make the claim, in absolute terms, that being fat doesn't have a negative impact on birth outcomes. We must be careful to clarify that stats and studies on things like PPH [postpartum haemorrhage] and shoulder dystocia haven't factored in comorbidities. However, because that's all the data there is, and it doesn't factor BMI away from other comorbidities, we can't say it doesn't.

AJ: Data would also likely be skewed by other aspects of care for fat folks, like fat folks are more likely to be induced.[2]

Amber: Exactly. It's tricky, because you can't say that there is no link, or that there is no increased risk, because the data shows that there is. However, the data is flawed, quite a lot of the time – because of the comorbidities, the differing treatment that fat people will receive, like not being able to access midwife-led units in some instances.

AJ: We still do have the stats that will show us that most of the fat or plus size women and people will have 'normal' pregnancy and delivery.

Amber: Yes, the increase of risk, again, is tricky. Because it gets reported as twice, three or four times more risk, but then you are talking about an extremely small risk.[3] For fat folks, yeah, it's doubled, but that is not reflective of the absolute risk.

AJ: Yep, you cannot argue that the risk hasn't doubled, but it's not now definitely going to happen.

---

2   www.nicswell.co.uk/health-news/obese-mums-more-likely-to-be-induced
3   https://maternityaudit.org.uk/FilesUploaded/NMPA%20BMI%20Over%2030%20Report.pdf

Amber: Yes, higher risk doesn't mean high risk! If someone says, 'You are high risk', that sounds like it's likely, as if it's more likely to happen than not. The rate of stillbirth, for example, does double from 3/1000 in women with a BMI of 18.5–24.9 to 6/1000 when BMI is 40+. This data does not consider variation of treatment from HCPs, restriction in birth choices, comorbidities etc., as we were discussing earlier. So, saying to service users with a BMI of 40+ that you are high risk of stillbirth because of your BMI isn't strictly true. You are more likely, you are twice as likely, to experience stillbirth if your BMI is over 40 than if your BMI is between 18.5 and 24.9, but that absolute risk is still a 0.06 per cent chance. It also treats everyone with a BMI of 40+ as one homogenous group. It doesn't factor in folks who have gestational diabetes, or folks with other pre-existing conditions or complications; 40+ is also a wide net in terms of BMI. Folks with a BMI of 41 are lumped in with folks with pre-existing conditions, or BMIs of 60+. It's not accurate to deal with statistics from such a large cohort with such varying experiences and access to treatment and care.

I think it's quite a lot to ask for service users to be able to find this data, interpret it and understand the flaws in that data and make decisions about their care based on sweeping statements that we see all too often, including 'You're high risk for your baby to die because of your BMI.' It's a big ask of me, and the highest qualification I have is a maths A Level!

AJ: Oh, don't sell that short, that is very impressive! A maths A Level! I could only dream!

Amber: Oh, I am proud of it, and I am really pleased that I have this basis of knowledge that when I work on or look at data sets, I see it through possibly slightly more informed eyes than most laypeople. Because what happens when a new stat comes out that fat people are twice as likely to experience stillbirth? That goes through many distillations and gets rolled out across trusts and down to an individual level to healthcare staff...and do they lead with the 'it's still less than a 1 per cent chance' or do they lead with 'twice as likely therefore high risk'? There is a lot more nuance to it than that, and it seems drastically unfair that your average punter turns up with a baby in their belly and they are told, 'You are high risk', and the fear of stillbirth is thrust on them in what we could fairly describe as disingenuous representation at best. I suppose it is just inherent fat bias within the healthcare system that so much autonomy and choice is taken from fat folks under the guise of 'high risk'.

It's not restricted just to fat people either; everyone I know who has had a baby has a story to tell. How they were belittled, how they weren't listened to or how they were disbelieved. I try to hold that in the back of my mind, too; it isn't all down to size. Can't say it's comforting, but it is important to remember it is not just fat folks being treated poorly!

AJ: So, as the founder of an incredibly successful and such a valuable, desperately needed community that is Big Birthas, what is it that people are coming to Big Birthas for?

Amber: People usually find us when they are looking for ideas on where to find maternity clothes! That is how most people enter the website or into the groups is when they are looking for 'what brands make maternity clothes for fat people?' They often aren't looking for information or statistics on fat birth or studies etc.; they are looking for the practical information about being fat and pregnant. Most people are looking for where can they get a good maternity bra or a maternity coat. They might find us when they are looking for information on slings and carriers for fat parents, but the articles or subjects that get me the biggest hits are the ones about clothes and other items in that general area. I thought the community would want the data, because that is what I wanted, but not everyone is Googling 'what is my risk of miscarriage because I am fat?'

AJ: I think this is important because no one is saying that finding clothes is the most pressing disparity for fat folks by a long stretch, but it is that tangible and relatable experience of how your choices and accessibility are restricted as you move up through the sizing. Most fat folks know that feeling of getting up and out to the high street or shopping centre and finding nothing in your size. I remember that from when I was a teenager, and I couldn't get clothes from the same shops as my cohort because they didn't carry above a size 16/18. That feeling of wishing you could wilfully shrink yourself so that you could at least get an item of clothing that was in the style of the latest fashion to, you know, experience that as a teenager where conformity is valued so highly, but having to settle for a jacket from the Army and Navy (I actually loved that coat in the end, but that's beside the point) because no one makes puffer jackets and stocks them in sizes above an 18 on the high street.

Amber: It is also how you present yourself to the wider world, every day. It is important that you are comfortable and feel good about yourself, and clothing and fashion can be an incredibly validating and self-esteem-boosting route to feeling good!

AJ: Erg, and when you do find the stores that do carry those sizes you are attacked at all angles from stripes and plaid, butterflies and slogan t-shirts that cost more than the t-shirts up the road in the store that only makes them to a size 20.

Amber: Not everyone wants an empire-line dress covered in butterflies to really signal femininity, and nor are we obsessed with making ourselves appear as small as possible!

AJ: Why is it always fucking butterflies?!

Amber: Ha ha, it's probably a metaphor for the skinny person inside our fat cocoons waiting to get out!!

AJ: It's the insistence that fat folks need to work harder to present femininity as well, I think. Being fat already moves you away from our society and culture's ideals of femininity: dainty, small, meek, quiet and covered in fucking butterflies.

Amber: Oh, and nothing that hugs your curves either! 'Here is a tent with butterflies on it... We don't want to show your fat body, so make sure it's all-flowing, non-hugging fabrics and cuts too.'

So that was my realization, that people are so frustrated with the lack of options in what becomes a very pressing need – we need to be clothed, right? So if people are finding the community through these routes, then I am all for it. I was quite lucky because the style of clothes that I tend to wear already lent themselves to my growing pregnant body. I lost weight in pregnancy, like you, and so I was able to get the same style of dresses I had always worn and just size up to accommodate my growing bump. However, if you are someone who wears jeans a lot, you are really going to struggle to find maternity jeans in these sizes.

AJ: The journey of finding jeans for fat bodies, period, is difficult enough let alone finding maternity ones.

Amber: Exactly, so I wrote an article about how to adapt mainstream fashion and what to look for in types of clothing that means you could wear it throughout pregnancy and beyond. Looking back 10–12 years ago when I was first pregnant, this was a necessity for me – there weren't any specific plus size maternity clothing brands. They just didn't exist. Plus size maternity wear is a niche within a niche. On the high street specifically, forget about it! It's hard enough to get decent clothes for fat people on the high street as it is.

AJ: I didn't do much clothes shopping when I was pregnant with Emma, but when I was pregnant with Izzy, the only store that carried a maternity range that went up to my size was Peacocks; sometimes I might find one or two pieces in New Look, but it was a gamble.

Amber: I think their standard range goes up to a 22/24, so maybe their maternity range does too.

AJ: Other brands like H&M that do in-store maternity ranges were just a no-go. I remember trying on a pair of jeans when I was early on in pregnancy with Emma, and I picked up a size 24 and they wouldn't go over my shins! I was smaller then than I am now, although my brain hasn't caught up that I am nearly 2.5 stones lighter than I was six months or so ago, so maybe I am about the same size as I was then, and a size 24 should be about right for me, especially as these were the style of maternity jeans with the stretchy panels in the pockets!

Amber: Love those! Very comfortable and practical!

AJ: I bought a pair of brown cords from the maternity section of Top Shop when I was about 16 because they were in the sale, they were my size, and they were comfortable!

Amber: Absolutely.

AJ: I am not surprised that looking for clothing is how many people could find communities like Big Birthas.

Amber: I do think there is an element, especially in your first pregnancy, where you go along to your appointments and you are told, 'You are high risk' and so you aren't looking to 'upset the apple cart' or 'buck the system'. You are being told by a professional that you are high risk, and you follow what they tell you. So they may come looking for information on bras and then see discussions or threads about someone else who is also being told they are high risk for stillbirth or death. As they read more they realize that they are not alone. They might see a thread of someone else's where they are talking about how they have been told they can't have a water birth, and other members who have had a water birth are sharing their experiences and talking about our right to give birth in a setting of our choosing.

They might then come to realize that they can say 'no' to these offers or interventions. They can ask for more information or more time to make their decisions.

A lot of people come with a fair amount of guilt and shame. A lot of people come from the base line of 'I probably shouldn't be pregnant because I am so fat.' That comes from society, from media, from family and medics. It is this general message of 'you are a bad person to have got to this point'. I've been in that exact position, too; time was ticking by, and I was 32 or so and starting to think, 'We need to think about having a baby now otherwise time will run out!' I was very aware I wasn't in peak physical fitness – but then I've never been in peak physical fitness!

AJ: Most people haven't been in peak physical fitness, regardless of body size!

Amber: It was just another barrier to our choices. There is already so much to consider when wanting to start or grow your family: do we have the money? The space? Are we prepared for the loss of income that often comes with poor maternity or paternity leave packages and support? Is our relationship stable? You know going through this process takes a toll on people's relationships, if they are coupled, of course. Many pregnancies happen without these considerations, obviously, but in these discussions before pregnancy we were considering so many variables, it was exhausting. Entering these systems and appointments then started from a place of 'Oh yeah, hi, I am pregnant, and I know my BMI isn't ideal...' already prepared for that to be a problem. But if I'd waited until some future date when I would magically be in better physical shape, it wouldn't happen at all, or I'd be old enough for that to be a concern instead! As with all things, there's a balance to be reached. Finding that balance in peer-to-peer communities can be difficult, too. Because we are not healthcare professionals, it's in our ground rules that we don't advise or give recommendations. Us telling people who join and ask if anyone else has decided to go for an elective caesarean birth that 'you should have a home birth', or women who have decided they don't want to breastfeed that they should breastfeed is just as bad as the HCP telling folks that they can't have a home birth – although we may ask people quietly behind the scenes to rephrase their words or think about the impact of their words on others, but in the four to five years we have been running, we have never had to kick anybody out of the Facebook group; it is such an incredible and wonderful community.

AJ: That is rare for parenting and pregnancy groups, let me tell ya!

Amber: It is! I am so proud of the community that we have created in Big Birthas. It is a community that is so needed, because it can feel so isolated to be fat and pregnant. We can't see another fat pregnant person in public and go over gushing, 'We are both fat and pregnant, let's be friends!' There are experiences of fat shaming or size bias that we experience that people who are not fat will not understand, or they won't understand why we are so nervous about being weighed, or worried about attending another scan because at the last scan they got annoyed and pushed the wand so hard into our tummy it was uncomfortable. Big Birthas provides that space where people do understand; they don't think you are just imagining things or being sensitive (or worse, that it's justified!) – and we've likely experienced it, or similar, ourselves.

AJ: In my experience as well, fat folks tend to be a bit more...guarded in discussing their health or their healthcare. I have written about my experience with my gallbladder already, and I know you know most of that tale because I would call you up knowing that what I needed was to speak to a fellow fatty who knew what these experiences of fat bias felt like. I didn't want to have those conversations with straight-sized people who have never experienced fatphobia in healthcare settings before because you find yourself almost...justifying why it's bad that they assumed it was all your fat's fault. We are more guarded because of our experiences of being dismissed and prescribed WeightWatchers, this experience of being diagnosed as fat.

Amber: We know we are fat as well! It's often delivered in a very quiet and gentle way, 'you may not know this' kind of vibe, 'but your BMI is high...'

AJ: Yeah I always want to say, 'Yeah, I know I am fat, I live everyday not fitting in, physically fitting into spaces or spaces not expecting me to be there, or brands not making clothes big enough for me so I can't join in with these fashion trends, random people coming up to me to talk about my body, service folks commenting on my food order or whatever, like, I am well aware I am fat. However, I don't think that is the main factor of my health, or a major factor in my current health complaint or why I am here.'

Amber: Yes, I don't think my ingrown toenail or broken bone is related to my fatness.

AJ: Right? So finding a community where we can say 'I'm not sure about taking the GTT [Glucose Tolerance Test] because the only risk factor is my BMI and I have been monitoring my BGL [blood sugar level] at home and it's all fine and I would rather continue monitoring this at home so it's immediate and more accurate of my actual food intake and exercise levels compared to the GTT', for example, finding that space, which might be the only space where we feel that we can have such discussions away from the insistence that fat bodies are ticking time bombs of risk and away from the 'because of your BMI you have to...' or 'because of your BMI you can't...' assertions of many (although not all) HCPs.

Amber: The absolute revelation for some people, it was for me, is that you can say 'no'. I think back to a lot of my experiences in my first pregnancy and now that I know that these 'offers' of induction, or whatever, it feels very different because they don't make it sound like an offer. People do come along to Big Birthas saying, 'I quite fancy a home birth' or the like and go on to say, 'but I've been told I am not allowed to' or 'I have been told I have to be induced' etc. So

121

when someone lets them know that these are all offers of treatment and you can decline their offer, you can take your time to consider and decide, it is often revelatory to them.

AJ: I wonder, if you surmise, as I often do, that...erm, what's the most diplomatic way to say this...

Amber: Don't worry about being diplomatic for me, ha ha!

AJ: Well, I've either got to figure it out now or later when I am typing this up!

Amber: Shall I try?

AJ: Yeah, go on...

Amber: Because we are fat, we must be stupid?

AJ: *Yes!* Ha ha, oh my god I might just type it exactly like that...[and I did].

Amber: Go for it, I think the thought process might be 'to have got to the size we are, we must be so stupid as to not realize how that has happened. Therefore how can we *possibly* be expected to make the right decisions about our pregnancy or birth?'

AJ: Hmmm, yes, if you aren't switched on enough or aware enough to not get fat, then how can you be trusted to make the right calls about your pregnancy or baby? You clearly don't know how to be healthy already, so why would we trust you now?

Amber: It feels more like a betrayal when it is a fat HCP too.

AJ: Oh absolutely, I remember the midwife who laughed at me when I said I wanted a water birth, she was fat! I remember thinking shouldn't there be some kind of kinship here? Like we both know how it feels to exist in a larger than expected body and how it affects our day-to-day lives, so it made it even worse that she was laughing at my birth choices.

Amber: I don't know if it is a defensive kind of position because I have been seen by fat medics who have been more fatphobic than straight-sized ones and, of course, I've seen fat medics who have been fabulous and straight-sized ones who have been horrifically awful.

You can, of course, request a different HCP, but finding a fat-positive one can be very difficult. Changing midwives or hospitals could disrupt your care as well. When I was pregnant I saw an obstetrician and she told me that on the basis of BMI I wouldn't be allowed to have a home birth. When I challenged that, and said that it was very concerning that she was falsely asserting that I had no say in where I gave birth, she got very defensive and asked, 'Oh, so you're the doctor now, are you?' It's not that I wanted to purposefully be awkward, but having your HCP say to you 'you can't do this' when you know that it is your body, your baby, your choice, really just destroys all that trust and ability to reason that they have your best interests at heart. You can't look out for people in this manner by coercing them and providing false information. I got a really shitty summary letter after that appointment that just angered me as well.

AJ: Oh this is one of your letters I haven't seen maybe!

Amber: Maybe we should put some in the book!

AJ: Maybe we should! Because although a lot of them will be a macro or a template, perhaps seeing these letters and how our fat is used to scapegoat, in some circumstances in writing, might help the point land? Like having 'maternal habitus' on all your scan paperwork.

Amber: I had to Google that when it was on my notes to find out what it means! I assume most service users would have to?! You go to your scan; they say, 'Oh yeah, everything is fine' and measuring this, that or the other, and you feel reassured. Then later, when you are looking over your notes, you see 'maternal habitus' all over the place.

AJ: There was a paper I saw that talked about how 'maternal habitus' isn't very well explained, and this leads to service users being of the opinion that there is blame, on them, for not being able to get an accurate scan. The team of this paper created a poster that basically explains what the ultrasound is and how it works, but most importantly they said that 'it does not depend on your size or body weight. It depends on whether you have the type of fat layer that spreads the sound beam. However, a thicker layer of fat is more likely to do this than a thin layer.'[4]

Amber: It also said it was important to note that when this occurs in patients with a low BMI, signalling it as 'body habitus' is not accurate, as someone with a normal or low BMI can still have the fat type that will obscure ultrasound:

> It may be better to phrase the report in terms of poor visualization due to 'poor echo quality' or 'poor echogenicity' rather than refer to 'obesity', 'body habitus' or 'high BMI'. This records the problem in the scan report for future reference but does not make reference to what may cause offence to the patient. It also covers the case where poor visualization is observed in a non-obese patient. Their BMI will be routinely recorded in their notes and in the case of a missed diagnosis all the relevant information is noted.
>
> It is important to understand that it is not obesity per se that is the cause. It is the type of fatty tissue that is the problem, namely non-uniform fatty tissue that has a matrix of both dense and less dense fat within it. Poor image quality may be seen in someone with a low BMI and a thin layer of such tissue, or perfectly clear images may be seen in someone with a higher BMI. Some people have this

---

4   www.ncbi.nlm.nih.gov/pmc/articles/PMC5105361

tissue type, some do not. This is a cause of misunderstanding amongst those being scanned.[5]

AJ: Doesn't sound accurate to label it as 'habitus' in any circumstance then? Because if it is not the size or shape of someone's body that leads to the inaccurate scan, it is the fat layer that can be present regardless of BMI, although it is more likely in folks with a higher BMI. Do we think that litigation is a factor, too?

Amber: Oh definitely. 'Anything goes wrong, we're not at fault here; it's all on you, you great fat blob.'

AJ: Maybe not in so many words, but it certainly seems to be on *a lot* of people's notes or letters. It was on my gallstone ultrasound report as well. Even though the tech, at the time, said he was able to get good measurements and good clear pictures for the report.

Amber: I find it particularly galling when they've literally just told you they got everything they needed...then write that imaging was sub-optimal. Either you could see everything fine, or you couldn't.

AJ: It doesn't promote trust or give reassurance, does it?

Amber: No, and when you have fat folks who have already absorbed guilt, shame and blame that their health and healthcare access are compromised by BMI, for years in some circumstances, adding another reason for us to blame our bodies, when it might not be our size or BMI that is causing the obstruction to clear imaging, just further isolates folks from their HCPs. We also put so much stock on scan results. We see this often in the community where women and people are told, 'Based on your scan measurements, you are going to have an abnormally large baby.' Then, 'You'll have to be induced or have a caesarean' based on these scans. To have 'body habitus' or 'poor

5   www.ncbi.nlm.nih.gov/pmc/articles/PMC5105361

visibility due to BMI' on those scan results when they are basing their recommendations of induction or caesarean birth means it wasn't clear. They said they could see fine, then they said they couldn't, yet this supposedly poor info is enough to recommend an intervention that is otherwise not indicated? Well, which is it? Could you see or could you not see?! It's important that I know how accurate that information is. I would love to see research about the estimated weights of babies of people with varying BMIs. I am highly suspicious that they expect fat folks to have larger babies and so they subconsciously measure slightly more generously – which, once the numbers are all multiplied together, inflates those birthweight estimates simply because we are large.

AJ: Baby's weight is commonly overestimated in ultrasounds, we know this to be the case.[6]

Amber: It's not to say, as with BMI, these findings can't be used as part of a bigger picture to frame decisions surrounding risk and benefits of proposed interventions, but using 'large' or 'small' baby as a standalone reason might not be accurate. I have witnessed, often in Big Birthas, people were saying that their scan's estimation of baby's weight was way off. Or maybe it's because those estimates are more likely to be used to coerce us into more medicalized treatment that it seems more of a problem.

AJ: That certainly was the case for both of my pregnancies. They said that Izzy was well over 10lbs and recommended induction, which we did, and then they were born 8lbs 4oz! Then with Emma a few years later I had extra growth scans because of the previous diagnosis of GD [gestational diabetes], and they said she was on the 50th centile line every time I had a scan...she was 9lbs 2oz! Which, for clarity, is not the 50th centile estimation weight!

Remembering this also made me remember when I had Izzy and

6   www.ncbi.nlm.nih.gov/pmc/articles/PMC5810856

when I said they were 8lbs 4oz a lot of people would say, 'Oh such a healthy weight', and even negative things like, 'Well you aren't small so it would make sense that you had a large baby!'

Then when Prince George was born the following summer and weighed 8lbs 6oz I remember feeling so miffed as to why people weren't going on about what a big baby he was!

Amber: Well, Kate Middleton is straight-sized. So when straight-sized people have an 8lbs-odd baby that is celebrated as a lovely big, bouncy, healthy baby! But when we have an 8lbs + baby it's a fat fucker because we are fat fuckers!

AJ: It's funny, but it is sad, too. These assumptions of fat = bad are even being applied to my few days-old baby! What chance does that give us to raise them in a space of body neutrality let alone even radical body acceptance?

Amber: We put so, so much stock into these measurements and we make so many decisions and restrict so many options based on them, and they just aren't as accurate as they are hailed to be. I was offered extra scans and I was quite happy to have those because I viewed it as more opportunity to see the baby.

AJ: That was the same for me, in my first pregnancy. Absolutely I want to see my baby again, of course! They would always say the same thing – head and legs are measuring larger than the stomach – and I would offer to parade my family members, all with three-quarters of their height in their legs and our giant mushroom heads. That's just the way we are built – apart from my dad who, although he was incredibly leggy, could also wear child-sized hats in his 50s and 60s – he liked that, though, because there wasn't any VAT, and he would feel like he was winning!

Amber: Mine were 7lbs 6oz and 7lbs 12oz, despite the 'well over 10lbs' warnings we were given, and it just seems too common a story, from the community and outside it, that we make these decisions about induction or sweeps or any of the rest of it based purely on scans that don't seem to be accurate enough to use as the sole basis for inducing labour. It comes back to BMI again, though, in a roundabout way, as BMI also doesn't take into account where you wear your fat or how long your legs are or how heavy your head is.

AJ: Totally...you could have two people who weigh exactly the same but look very different based on height, muscle mass, breast size, head size – so many variables.

Amber: Conversely, my friend who is 5-foot nothing and of very average build was told all throughout pregnancy, 'Oh, your baby is small', and she would answer, 'Well, yes, of course, we are both small people with slight builds, it stands to reason that we wouldn't produce a giant.'

AJ: We have such a narrow view of what is too big and what is too small and what is healthy or at risk based on a calculation that doesn't take into consideration the naturally occurring variables of human beings!

Amber: Absolutely.

AJ: So people come to Big Birthas in search of practical information about clothes and other things and this is where, for some, this is the first look at people declining interventions or challenging the blanket statements of 'Your baby is at risk' or 'You are at risk' purely because of BMI...

Amber: It's about choice and control. Who should have the control and who has the power, and where should it rest?

AJ: Regardless of your BMI you are always in control and your autonomy and choice should always be centred in maternity and perinatal services. I don't think we could over-state that point.

Amber: That can be quite a revelation to people. We see it time and time again in the threads, comments and discussions, people saying, 'I didn't realize I could say "no"!?'

Yes! You are allowed to say 'no'! We are so lucky to have the NHS, that goes without saying, but when you go to the doctors or the midwife etc. and you don't actually hand over money there and then, it doesn't feel as if you are paying for it. So we have a unique experience on top of the English sensibilities of not making a fuss, being a good girl or a polite person combined with a feeling of not being in the driving seat, and that we must be grateful for this free treatment and service. Then they start to read the stats and the experiences of other folks, and for some, they then happen on their own internalized fatphobia.

AJ: That is a tough place to arrive at, isn't it? When we are confronted with our own internal bias or assumptions about our own selves. It can feel very much as if the ground has been whipped away from you. Our entire lives we have been told by the entire world that fat = bad. Coming face to face with that wee beasty in your mind and asking yourself, 'Who told me that?' is terrifying.

Amber: It is, but the release of guilt can be incredibly profound for people. Being able to look at the data and say, 'Oh, I am only marginally more likely to have a stillbirth based on my weight, and that data might be skewed because it is taking *everyone* with a BMI of over 40 (or the like), including people with underlying conditions and other factors, and I don't have any underlying conditions or any of the other predisposition factors, and even if I did, it's still only increasing by 0.02 per cent.'

We see people benefiting from having that space to share these concerns and their journeys with other people who have experienced it too. People have come in and their first post ever has been 'Am I selfish for becoming pregnant at my size?' or 'Am I crazy for thinking about trying to conceive at my size?' We get a lot of questions like this about home birth: 'Am I crazy?' 'Is it selfish?' 'Am I allowed?' Even folks who come and say, 'I've had 1/2/3/4 babies already and everything has always gone well, and I am considering staying at home for a multitude of reasons and I want to...' still with this assumption that they need permission because of their size to decide where they want to give birth.

AJ: This is where I often get so confused, because speak to any birth worker or HCP and they will agree that service users should be given the information that they need or want to make an informed decision on their birth choices, including place of birth. We know that it is protected in law, we know why those protections are essential in preserving the autonomy of pregnant people. Yet so many people come away from these appointments, classes or clinics having been given the impression that they are not in charge. What is being lost in translation for fat folks here? Does it relate to your eloquent and succinct: 'because you're fat you must be thick?' Because as you point out, many people approaching plus size or fat birth have already absorbed fatphobia and carry internalized fatphobia with them through this process and the rest of their lives.

Amber: I would, if I had a platform to speak to all fat people accessing care, want them to know that 'regardless of your BMI you are in control. Your BMI doesn't remove you of your autonomy.'

AJ: What, if anything, then, would you say to HCPs or birth workers on this subject?

Amber: I wrote a blog about 'How to be a plus size friendly professional'. It covers many things including assumptions and imagery – e.g., don't just have pictures of headless fat people, or fat people eating junk food on your posters and no positive imagery of people who look like us – we are allowed to look happy! We frequently do. Another aspect is that they feel as if they must tell us we are fat. People experience this at every healthcare interaction, this 'passing of information that you might not have been aware of' regarding their fatness. We are already aware that we exist in larger than expected bodies. If, at every point in your first interaction with us, your first answer to all our problems is 'you have a high BMI', then how is that going to grow trust? Enable fat folks, who society already sees as lazy and stupid, to self-advocate and work with HCPs in their pregnancy journey.

AJ: I think that is a really valid point that perhaps particularly straight-sized professional won't realize: that most of us have been diagnosed as fat before, many times. Before we have even conceived or gone to our first midwife appointment, a lot of us are expecting to be told fat = bad. Before we've even stepped through the doors of the clinic, we are anticipating size bias and fatphobia.

Amber: Yes, and I also say to professionals, please remember that this is your everyday. Seeing people and discussing their conceptions, pregnancies and birth, you do this day in, day out, and it becomes normalized. For the service user, this is anything but a normal day; this might be the first time they have attended a midwifery clinic, or this might be the first time that someone says to them, 'Your baby is at high risk of stillbirth because of your BMI.' It can be the single most important journey of our lives that we take. We will remember what you say to us for years, decades, in some instances. More than that, we will remember how you made us feel. If I had to distil it down to just one point, it is that you can ask someone in their 90s about their birth experience and they will remember, with accuracy, how they felt. They may not remember the exact wording, or the names or faces of the doctors or midwives, but they will remember how they felt.

AJ: It is fascinating, isn't it? I remember when I first started training to be a doula and one of the first things we did as mothers and gestational parents in a room together was talk about our births. I went home and told my nan about my day at training, and she told me about her births. I told someone else about what I was doing, and they told me about their births; someone overheard, and they joined in the conversation about their births. They weren't talking about the length of time from first to second stage (in most cases); they weren't talking about the sickness or scans or that one grumpy doctor. They were talking about how they felt, what they still feel when they close their eyes, or when they look at their babies.

My nan was diagnosed with Alzheimer's around that time, and anyone who's loved or cared for someone with Alzheimer's will tell you, they retell certain stories over and over again. One of my nan's staples was her birth stories – how they made her feel stupid because she had been picking up her eldest child when pregnant with her second. How they chastised her for working up until she was hospitalized with her second, my dad. She was just shy of a century when she passed, and she told those stories until the day she died. Well that's not true, she told those stories until the day Alzheimer's took her voice from her.

Amber: It's not fair to expect a platinum standard of healthcare 24/7 from doctors, nurses or midwives, because they are human beings. Coming into work after being kept up by their own babies or children, or caring for their elders and loved ones, on top of working in a profession that is underpaid, understaffed and wards and clinics that don't have the right resources. They are human beings; of course there will be the odd slip or misstep, it's not about demanding perfection. But it is about demanding humanizing and individualized treatment, regardless of body size. Sometimes it's not about the words they use, it's about the distrust that their treatment causes. Or the callous way in which we are spoken to that causes these experiences to get stuck on repeat in our heads. Birth experiences are seldom something that get deleted in a defrag years later – it sticks! So remember how important this experience is to us. Remember how long it is likely to stay with us.

AJ: What else haven't we said that needs to be said, Amber?

Amber: If you Google 'fertility symbols' or 'carvings like fertility god-desses' statues' or historical 'mother' pieces – they are usually fat. These totemic sculptures from ancient civilizations are, usually, volup-tuous: big thighs, big bums, big bellies, big boobs! Where did that change? When did that stop? We have this modern idea of health and fertility as straight sized. If these artefacts are showing us what fer-tility goddesses look like, and if this is what pregnancy and fertility looks like, then hell, I am there!

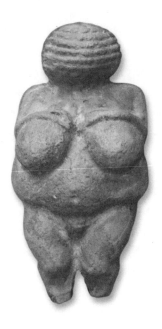

CHAPTER 9

Gestational Diabetes

This is a topic that is close to my heart – having been diagnosed with GDM (gestational diabetes mellitus, often shortened to GDM/GD) in the 24th week of my first pregnancy, having a BMI that is lower than my current BMI (couldn't tell you what it was back then; I've blocked a lot of it out, to be frank). I was offered an oral Glucose Tolerance Test (OGTT, often shortened to GTT) at my local hospital. I was asked to fast for 10 hours and then present myself to one of the maternity wards. Feeling a little nauseated and tired at best, I took my fat ass up there and waited to have my Lucozade. For anyone who hasn't had the pleasure, the GTT is often carried out by fasting overnight and then having bloods drawn before and after drinking Lucozade (although in some trusts you are offered specific foods rather than Lucozade).

Before we go any further, it's important that I say this to you if you have been diagnosed with GD: it's not your fault. Service users are often told that the reason they are being referred or offered testing for GD is because they have one of the following risk factors:[1]

- BMI over 30
- Previously had a baby who weighed 4.5kg (10lbs) or more at birth
- Previously diagnosed with GD
- One of their parents or siblings has diabetes

---

1   www.nhs.uk/conditions/gestational-diabetes

- They are of South Asian, Black, African-Caribbean or Middle Eastern origin (even if they were born in the UK).

It can be assumed by these service users that there is blame for their increased likelihood to develop GD. It is important that we look at the study that Deborah Hughes highlights in her book for AIMS (Association for Improvements in the Maternity Services), *Gestational Diabetes:*[2] 'Nevertheless, nearly half of women diagnosed with GDM do not have any of these risks factors and many that do have them do not develop GDM.'

It is also important to discuss increased risk versus absolute risk. For example, if someone is told their risk doubles, this sounds scary! But, as Dr Sara Wickham writes in her 2014 book *Inducing Labour*:

> For the past few years, the reference most commonly used in the UK Documents was a paper by Hilder et al, published in 1998, which showed that the rate of perinatal death is at its lowest at about one in a thousand at 21 weeks, rising to about two in a thousand from 42 weeks. It was on the basis of this data that it was proposed that routinely offering induction of labour between 41 and 42 weeks might prevent the death of those additional one in a thousand babies. Some women were told that the risk to their baby doubled at this time, but I hope you can see from these figure that, while this statement was technically accurate, it might not have been the clearest way of discussing the situation with women.[3]

Moving from 1 in 1000 to 3 in 1000 is tripling. But it doesn't accurately represent the actual risk. It is true that the risk does triple, but it is still low. It rises from 0.1 per cent to 0.3 per cent.

From 'The influence of maternal BMI and gestational diabetes on

---

2   www.google.com/search?client=safari&rls=en&q=getational+diabetes+deborah+hug hes+aims&ie=UTF-8&oe=UTF-8, p.28.
3   www.sarawickham.com/iol, p.81.

pregnancy outcome' study,[4] the actual risk of developing GD looks very different:

- BMI 25 to <30: 6.74%
- BMI 30 to <35: 13.42%
- BMI 35 to <40: 12.79%
- BMI <40: 20%.

The Centers for Disease Control and Prevention (CDC) in the USA states that 'every year, 2%–10% of pregnancies in the United States are affected by gestational Diabetes'.[5] Diabetes UK states that GD 'occurs in 3–5% of pregnancies'.[6] So if the 'base risk' is 5 per cent (as an average across these figures), then it is arguably factual that someone with a BMI of 35 to 40 has around a three times greater risk than at the national levels. However, this doesn't mean that if the service user had a BMI of <25 that they would not have been diagnosed with GD.

It is also worth considering that those who exist in larger bodies are screened more often for GD as well as those who are of South Asian, Black or Middle Eastern heritage, those who have had large babies previously, those previously diagnosed with GD, and those whose immediate relatives have diabetes.

It also doesn't tell us how many folks are 'border line' and treated as if they are gestationally diabetic as a 'precaution'. To use my fat self again as an example, in my second pregnancy, having been diagnosed through a GTT in my first pregnancy and finding that that restricted my birth choices to a level that caused me trauma, I balanced the risks of the GTT and its knock-on effects with the risk of undiagnosed GD. I decided that to mitigate the risks of undiagnosed GD, I would monitor my blood glucose levels (BGLs) at home. I double-checked the current NICE (National Institute for Health and Care Excellence) guidelines for BGLs, and set about monitoring them from early on in pregnancy. Being able to afford a blood glucose monitor, test strips

---

4   https://pubmed.ncbi.nlm.nih.gov/25796512
5   www.cdc.gov/diabetes/basics/gestational.html
6   www.diabetes.co.uk/gestational-Diabetes.html

and lancets isn't a privilege that all pregnant people have. However, it did afford me with real-time information on my BGL. It was accurate about my dietary and exercise habits as well as being immediate! This enabled me to eliminate the risk of undiagnosed GD while not risking the 'false positives' or inaccurate diagnosis that can occur.

A study into a false positive 1-hour glucose challenge test and adverse perinatal outcomes[7] showed a risk of false positives to be around 9 per cent: 164 participants out of 1825 were identified as false positive, and 50 out of 1825 were categorized as GD, which is roughly a 3 per cent rate. It was therefore over three times more likely, in this study at least, that folks were misdiagnosed as having GD than having GD. Or 3 per cent versus 9 per cent. Roughly.

The article concludes that 'a false-positive is an independent risk factor for adverse perinatal outcomes'. Additionally, 'The false-positive GCT [glucose challenge test] cohort on average was older, of high parity, had a higher body mass index, and more frequently had chronic hypertension, sickle cell trait, and elevated mid-trimester human chorionic gonadotropin levels...macrosomia [big baby] greater than 4500g...antenatal death...shoulder dystocia...endometritis...and caesarean delivery.'[8]

Having been told I was gestationally diabetic I was sent to a specialist midwifery clinic for folks with GD. We were sat in a specific part of the waiting room, next to the vending machines, for added satire. We were also weighed at clinic to make sure we weren't gaining more weight. When my weight continued to go down in my first and second trimester, I was praised! 'Well done, you must have really changed your eating habits!' Yeah, no shit! I was scared to eat because the time spent in GD clinics was largely obsessed with having grown-ass people point to pictures on print-outs of what they thought was the 'correct' size portion of mashed potato, and being scared stiff about my baby dying because I have GD, because I am fat.

Having made it through to my 35th week I tottered into my

7   https://pubmed.ncbi.nlm.nih.gov/14704259
8   https://pubmed.ncbi.nlm.nih.gov/14704259

consultant appointment, I thought to discuss my birth plans and options. However, I was immediately greeted with, 'Your weight is lower than your last appointment again, well done. So we're going to go ahead and schedule you for induction on 39 weeks.' Being a fresh-faced first-time parent at the age of 23 I didn't know then what I know now (that you can decline their offers of intervention) and agreed. After three days of pessaries and drips I texted Adam asking him to bring some Tums when he came back in the morning because I kept having these tummy aches come and go, like, every 10–15 minutes – I did say I was fresh-faced, eh? When Adam turned up in the morning, he found a midwife behind the curtain breaking my waters as I had been contracting all night (apparently I thought I had a stomach ache!). Shortly after, we were all transferred to a delivery room. I was fitted with the standard practice intravenous medications for GD labours: a sliding-scale glucose drip (so that they can control your BGL, given that you aren't eating) in one hand and my Syntocinon (which makes the uterus contract) drip in the other. Two sensors were then placed on my bump, and we were told the anaesthetist would be in shortly to fit my epidural. Scared and unable to move at all, both my hands plugged in and the straps across my belly moving and people getting cross when I tried to move because the sensor couldn't get baby's heartbeat, I plumped for staying as still and as small as possible. When the very tall and dashing anaesthetist did come in, I greeted him by removing the gas and air from my face long enough to throw up on his shoes, which he so charmingly shook off (both figuratively and physically). After he left, I don't remember much. I remember flashes like trying to get up and being told to stay still and, 'Stop screaming, you'll scare other people in the ward, and you are wasting your energy!' I also remember asking where the baby was, despite my current labouring. Mostly I remember the look in Adam's eyes when the midwife asked him to hit the big red button above my head and about eight people came rushing in. But a few minutes, or it could have been a few hours later, I wasn't really there at this point, and Izzy was in my arms.

Evidently, as I was told in the postnatal ward, my baby's heart rate was dropping a bit and it was just best to just get baby out as soon as they could.

In complete contrast, as I helped Emma up and out of the water in my living room with my doula, Adam and a lone midwife sitting on her hands across the room, I remember every moment – the laughter when my doula pointed out I had done most of my labours next to my fridge (a cold, tiled floor on that very hot July day), and how I should have told them the reason for my wanting a home birth was 'fatty can't leave the fridge'. I remember Adam gently sighing when I asked him to fill up the pool, but he had to do that without leaving my side. I also remember the feeling of that warm water enveloping me in its safe and weightless embrace.

My consultant appointment at 35 weeks with Emma went slightly differently, despite it being the very same consultant, same hospital and, in fact, the very same office. I went prepared with my print-outs and notes on my phone to remind me of what I wanted to say. When I said, 'My baby will be born at home into the water', she drew breath. She went to say something, and I leaned forward, ready...but she stopped short, started looking through my notes and eventually said, 'Yeah, okay...' I waited for the 'but'...however, when she continued, she said, 'It's your second baby, you've been monitoring your own BGL and that's all been fine, you did have a PPH [postpartum haemorrhage] in your first labours, but you were induced early and you were on your back, so maybe at home in the water...yeah...okay fine.' Feeling triumphant and free I went home and texted my doula 'Drop the pool over baby, we're good to go!'

In the last few weeks, like many people, I experienced difficulty with maintaining my blood sugar levels. In both of my pregnancies it was my fasting/morning numbers that were creeping up. Commonly referred to as the 'dawn phenomenon', the cause isn't clear. Some consider the effects of changing hormones as we sleep; others think this is a natural reaction to not having eaten for many hours so the body dumps stored sugars and therefore the blood glucose level rises. Whatever the cause, the way I found to manage this was to have a pint of water with a few Brazil nuts and a few diced cubes of cheese.

This combination of fats and proteins seemed to stem the effects of the dawn phenomenon for me and the many other people on the groups who can attest to this. I asked my midwife if I could have an appointment with the diabetic midwife to get some other ideas on meals and snack suggestions as, in the final stages, as some people do, I was experiencing higher BGLs. She obliged, and a few days later the GD midwife called me. At first she was confused as she couldn't find my GTT result so didn't know how or why I was on her workload. Once I had brought her up to speed, she let me know that the overall message was to eat less, and move more.

There are many websites, books, blogs, social media accounts and more dedicated to sharing ideas for GD meals that may help folks with diet-controlled GD keep their BGL inside the parameters, so I won't waste time doing this here. However, I will share my lived experience over two gestational diabetic pregnancies – one where I injected insulin in the final few weeks and one where I remained diet-controlled.

Before I talk a bit more about my experience, I want to make it absolutely crystal clear that remaining diet-controlled isn't always in your control. Taking a page from the 'diet and health morality' playbook, remaining diet-controlled is often lauded as the best. This means that you have stopped eating all the bad shit and you've got your butt up off the sofa for that post-meal walk every time, right? Not always. If your BGL won't behave no matter what steps you take to try and mitigate the circumstances, please know – it's not your fault. It's not because of how big you are, or because of any other factor within your control. Remember: 'Nevertheless, nearly half of women diagnosed with GDM do not have any of these risk factors and many that do have them do not develop GDM.'[9]

From person to person, week to week, and even day by day, what causes your sugars to peak may change. It's easy to get frustrated and confused, especially as the advice on diet can often be lacking. I remember having a cry (standard) at the midwife appointment

---

9   https://shop.aims.org.uk/products/gestational-diabetes, p.69.

because I was so hungry in the mornings: I couldn't stomach any more eggs, and all kinds of bread I could find were making me feel sick; even porridge was betraying me, and I was told to eat one Weetabix for breakfast. I was 36 weeks pregnant – one Weetabix wasn't going to touch the sides. I found out about three days after this appointment through support groups, and trial and error, that if I also had a protein shake with my porridge, this gave my body the extra protein and fat (full fat milk) to help break down the carbohydrates, so I could have porridge again.

It's also a common and understandable mistake that folks assume that any kind of diet means a low fat diet. So when we phrase dietary restrictions as a GD *diet*, it's understandable that consciously or unconsciously many of us will be reaching for the low fat or reduced fat options. However, these can often contain more sugar and/or carbohydrates than the 'full fat' version, and can cause spikes in BGL. I found this out the hard way with a low fat yoghurt that I had purchased to put on some mixed berries! Queue the hypo. In my second pregnancy I would have added a protein full fat yoghurt and a few berries, and sometimes I would also have oats with them. No hypo. This coupling of foods was a game-changer for me. Realizing that processing the glucose and carbohydrates was easier for my body when it had sufficient fibre, fat and protein to do so meant I was better able to predict what my body might need. From my first pregnancy I was used to estimating the insulin injection amount, so I surmised a not entirely dissimilar calculation: Xg of carbs of sugar = Yg of protein/fat/fibre. It is obviously not an exact science, but it was also a handy prompt to have a quick check over my plate and consider the building blocks of my meal, and if it was going to give my body the best chance at breaking down the carbohydrates and sugars.

In 2012, when I was pregnant for the first time, my BMI was absolutely lower than when I was pregnant for the second time in 2015. During my first pregnancy I was unable to control my blood glucose levels and was injecting insulin by week 28. I was diet-controlled throughout my second pregnancy, when I was fatter. One of the reasons I expect that I was able to diet-control the second time round and not the first was the access to information I had. I had a two-year-old and loads of parent friends, some of whom had had GD during their pregnancies, and they were able to recommend meal ideas and Facebook groups to find support! It was in those communities that I found out about the Brewer Diet, coupling foods, the importance of full fat options, a snack before bedtime to help with morning fasting numbers, and much more. These communities are often invaluable resources where you can find someone else who understands how it feels to have a crushing craving for just one Haribo Tangfastic (the sour cherries, if you must know), but reluctantly accepting that half of a sniff will be enough to send your BGL over 10 and you to bed for the rest of the day. Gestational Diabetes UK also has huge resources offering diet and meal ideas. I have made plenty of these dinners in my two pregnancies and one or two are still in the rotation (curried tikka salmon and roasted chickpea salad with wholemeal pittas [chef's kiss]).

Gestational Diabetes UK's 8 Golden Rules to eating are useful in an experience that is often confusing, and help simplify the information to eight succinct points:

1. Eat little and often.

2. 'Pair' foods (e.g., protein and carbs).

3. Eat high protein.

4. Eat good, natural fats.

5. Eat low amounts of unrefined complex starchy carbohydrates at every meal.

6. Bulk up meals with lots of vegetables and salad.

7. Drink plenty of water.

8. Go for a stroll.

Eating little and often is what a lot of pregnant people will do naturally. This might be due to the lack of space in the later stages of pregnancy or sickness or nausea in the early stages. For folks with GD, eating little and often may help control BGL within the required parameters. Becoming too scared to eat through fear of eating the wrong thing is also a common experience of people with GD. The body can then release stored sugars to help even out the BGL, causing a high BGL despite not eating. This, in turn, can cause even more frustration and fear. Similarly, avoiding all carbs is a conclusion that many people, somewhat understandably, arrive at to combat their carb intolerance. Carbs are vital for energy, something in high demand when creating an entire human being. If you aren't eating enough carbs, the body will break down fat in your body for energy, which can lead to ketosis: everybody makes ketones and they are usually completely metabolized. However, when the body is burning fat stores for energy, this process causes an increase in ketone production, called ketosis. Usually detected via a urine dipstick test, it's common for pregnant folks to have ketones in their urine. However, if they are persistent, even after eating and drinking well, or a very high reading is observed, you may be advised to eat little and often and to make sure you are hydrated. You may also be invited to have an intravenous drip with fluids to help 'flush' the ketones from your system and to restore regular function. This is because 'A number of clinical studies have proved that high ketone bodies in women with GDM are associated with various adverse pregnancy outcomes.'[10]

Reducing or regulating BGLs through physical activity doesn't have to look like nauseating Instagram-filtered pregnancy workouts. I found timing the dog walk after my largest meal of the day (lunch) helped my BGL fall faster than if I didn't go for a walk. It is important to balance this with the increased rest that you are likely to need when baking a human from scratch. A study of a small group in Japan showed a correlation between lower BGL and more steps walked. It concluded that 'Simple walking for light intensity physical activity is effective for controlling the BGL in pregnant women with GDM.

---

10   www.ncbi.nlm.nih.gov/pmc/articles/PMC7701151, p.4586.

We recommend that pregnant women with GDM should walk a minimum of 6000 steps a day.'[11]

If walking isn't suitable for you, other actives such as swimming or a pregnancy aerobics class might be beneficial. If, like me, you find swimming up and down a pool to be a drag when you could be perfecting your bombing or being absolutely feral diving under and emulating dolphins and whales, dancing is a fantastic alternative – in the nightclub, if you so choose. I've found nothing more freeing or liberating than dancing to the cheesiest, most-likely-to-be-deleted-from-my-public-Spotify-playlist-worthy tunes to be cathartic for both body and soul. Tommy's, the baby loss charity, adds: 'As a general rule, you should still be able to hold a conversation as you exercise. If you become breathless, you're probably pushing yourself too hard. Keep exercise moderate, with rest periods, so that you do not become exhausted.'[12]

---

11 www.ncbi.nlm.nih.gov/pmc/articles/PMC6174974, p.1731.
12 www.tommys.org/pregnancy-information/pregnancy-complications/gestational-diabetes/staying-active-gestational-diabetes

CHAPTER 10

Water Birth

It came as no surprise, to anyone who knows me, that I wanted a water birth. I was a water baby, albeit not born into water the way in which water babies are usually characterized. In fact, I was born six weeks early and weighed just over 4lbs. 'We took the clothes off the dolly's back', my Nanny Win would say to me as she chased me clear of whatever hell I was raising under her feet. My love of water might have come from my dad, a fisherman who caught marlin in the Gulf of Mexico, sharks in the North Sea and often a hangover to match. When my dad died in 2020, we found he had more photographs of boats he'd owned or sailed in, fish that he had caught and sights he had seen from said boats than of people. Classic Bob.

Even though I learned at my dad's knee how to hook a worm, cast out, reel in and certainly how to swear like a sailor, I was never keen on swimming in the sea. The tide rising and falling could and has captivated me for hours, but swimming in it, not so much. I was keen, however, on jumping into swimming pools and soaking in baths or hot tubs. I can still see my mum's exacerbated and furrowed brow behind her raincoat and umbrella as I perfected my cannon balls and allowed her to time my breath-holding endeavours during the deluge at the caravan park's pool.

Ever since my mum ran me a warm bath to comfort me during my early menstruation, it has been one of the only things that provides relief. When pregnant with Izzy I had told the midwife I was considering a water birth on the basis that water provides me with such relief and comfort during menstruation. This was, as previously mentioned, met with a hearty snort of derision. When pregnant for a second time, I decided, as many do, that the risk of being denied a water birth before, during or after my labours wasn't a risk I was prepared to take. I chose to labour at home safe in the knowledge that my own, cannot be occupied, cannot not be cleaned, cannot be denied getting in the pool was going to be available for me to use.

Given the many benefits of labouring and birthing in water, it is a wonder why so many pregnant women and people find that they run into difficulty in accessing a pool. Whether your BMI is too high, your GD not controlled enough, your conception too medical or your age too advanced, there are no shortages of perceived incompatibilities with a water birth. Even if you or your baby aren't high risk, and your hospital trust has birth pools, it's not unusual to find many 'house-keeping' conflicts to access. From 'It hasn't been cleaned' to 'It's being used right now' or 'There isn't a water birth midwife available'; even 'We don't have sufficient staff to operate the winch in case of emergency evacuation from the water.' There is no shortage of reasons that the best-laid water birth plans of women and people often go astray.

We do know that water birth reduces the need for pain relief and use of epidural as well as a reduction in duration of first stages of labour.[1] I felt so safe in my little warm and inflatable den. I was protected, not from a sabre-toothed cat or anything equally prehistoric, but for the same reasons many mammals, where able, hunker down to nest in enclosed, warm and dark places. I, and many others, crave that too.

Amber Marshall's AIMS article ('High BMI waterbirth – Time for trusts to take the plunge?') has a wealth of information that will be invaluable for anyone in a bigger body, planning a water birth:

> The Winterton Report in 1992 recommended that all maternity services provide women with the option to labour and/or birth in water...
> Current Nice Guidance on intrapartum care for healthy women and babies expressly recommends caregivers 'Offer the woman the

---

1   www.cochranelibrary.com/cdsr/doi/10.1002/14651858.CD000111.pub3/epdf/abstract, p.1.

opportunity to labour in water for pain relief', yet in many cases, despite the absence of other risk factors, anyone with a BMI over 40 (or in some Trusts over 35) is automatically excluded from this option.

...no reasons for this arbitrary limit are given; a situation replicated across the UK, with many posts on pregnancy and parenting forums from frustrated women bearing witness to it. It is very difficult to find written justification, and since guidelines as these are the reference point for clinicians, it is unsurprising that refusal reasons given in consultations are often vague. Most seem to stem from:

- Manual handling assumptions
- Emergency evacuation concerns
- Perceived difficulty with fetal monitoring...

Aside from the automatic exclusion of anyone with a 40+ BMI, Salisbury NHS' Guide states 'women with a BMI of over 35 at booking should be informed that their suitability for labouring and or delivering in water will be individually assessed as to their ability to leave the pool'. Surely this should be extended to all prospective pool users? Not everyone with a BMI of 35+ is immobile, and not everyone with a BMI of 34 or less is agile. To make assumptions on someone's abilities, and then through that decide their care pathway solely based on a mathematical function of their height and weight, is absurd.[2]

Absurd at best, and harmful at worst. To assume that all service users with a BMI of under 30/35/40 (Warning: 'cut-offs' may vary) have the same access needs is a disservice to those service users, as well as the service users barred from water birth on the assumption of their mobility. Considering what we know and have discussed already about the inaccuracy of BMI to confirm or deny a person's health, we can suitably discharge the assumption that BMI also predicts a person's mobility. Individualized assessment seems to be the only way

---

2   www.aims.org.uk/journal/item/waterbirth-high-bmi

to accurately attest to someone's ability to manoeuvre, with support, themselves in and out of a birthing pool. I agree with Amber – absurd.

Health and safety, I hear you cry – this is 2023 after all. You'll be happy to hear that Amber's article confirms:

A report by the Health & Safety Executive (HSE) details the manual handling risks to midwives associated with birthing pools; which are largely due to poor ergonomics prompting poor posture in the midwife attending or from the midwife actively supporting the mother on entry/exit. However, the report goes on to give examples of good pool design to mitigate against these risks, which are not exclusive to the care of those with high BMIs.

This HSE report also looks at emergency evacuation: 'The two main methods reported for removing the mother from the pool in an emergency are a patient hoist (and sling) or a purpose designed lifting net...the hoist method was least preferred by midwives...however, for maternity units with limited numbers of midwives, the hoist method is preferred as a minimum of 4 staff would be required for the net method.'

The emergency evacuation scenario is probably the most often cited reason for denial of access; specifically, 'the hoist isn't strong enough'. But using BMI in this example is fallacious when a 5'6" woman weighing 15st 5lbs (BMI 34) is allowed to use the pool, yet a 5' woman weighing 13st 3lbs isn't (BMI 36). A hoist's safe working load is determined by weight, not BMI.

In any case, the RCOG Management of Women with Obesity in Pregnancy Guidelines recommends equipment is supplied with 'safe working loads up to 250kg' (i.e. sufficient for someone of 6'6" with a BMI of 62) and 'lifting and lateral transfer equipment' is specifically listed. So if we're following the rest of the guidelines which have been published for nearly a decade, why aren't suitable hoists routinely available?[3]

---

3   www.aims.org.uk/journal/item/waterbirth-high-bmi

These are the same guidelines that state that appropriately sized blood pressure cuffs and dignity wear be available for us, and those of us living in bigger bodies unfortunately know how often these provisions are not afforded to us.

After all of this, we of course come full circle, back to the beginning: how every conversation, discussion or plan of birth or labour, including where and how, is only ever the choice of the pregnant person, regardless of the trust's or hospital's guidelines or 'cut-offs'. Your BMI doesn't prevent you from having a water birth. As Amber says in her article:

> Of course, what Salisbury NHS Trust means is that women with a BMI above 40 'will not be *permitted* to labour or deliver in water on *their* premises'. I, and many others with a BMI of 40+ can conclusively prove that we are perfectly *able* to do so, but we sadly often have to put up a fight with our caregivers (and in many instances insist on a home birth) in order to achieve a water birth.[4]

Speaking of which…

---

4   www.aims.org.uk/journal/item/waterbirth-high-bmi

CHAPTER 11

Home Birth

Wanting a water birth isn't the only reason that fat folks may want to labour and birth at home.

There is no BMI caveat in the Department of Health's guidance *Maternity Matters: Choice, Access and Continuity of Care in a Safe Service*,[1] which confirms that the decision over place of birth, including the decision to give birth at home, is a 'national choice guarantee'. Nor is there a BMI limit on Article 8 of the human rights act that guarantees the right to private family life. Indeed in 2011, *Ternovszky v. Hungary* confirmed at the European Court of Human Rights confirmed that Home Birth is a European human right.[2] Although folks might, understandably, be under the impression that you need a home birth (water birth, opting out of induction etc.) 'signed off' or approved by a midwife or obstetrician, this is not the case.

Your healthcare team may want to meet with you to ensure that you have all the information you need to make an informed decision regarding your birth choices, but you certainly don't need their permission to birth your baby in your home. It is not illegal to give birth at home under any circumstances (consider how many people caught unaware by fast labours, unknown pregnancies, traffic jams, lack of ambulances and more would be convicted if this were the case). It is also not illegal to give birth without a midwife or medical professional present. Free birth (birthing without medical assistance)

---

1   http://familieslink.co.uk/download/july07/Maternity%20matters.pdf
2   https://www.internationalmidwives.org/assets/files/statement-files/2018/04/eng-home-birth14.pdf

is not illegal, despite many misinformed people attesting otherwise. The only requirement of expectant or new parents is to register the baby's birth. Other than that, you choose what services, appointments, interventions etc. you would like. This includes scans, all appointments, induction of labour – you name it. It's your body, your baby, your choice. You are also allowed to change healthcare provider and/ or hospital. If you think that changing midwife, health visitor, hospital or obstetrician might be better for you, you are always within your right to do so. If any HCP continues to treat you once you have withdrawn your consent to be treated by them, that is assault.

As we covered in Chapter 10 on water birth, hospitals, trusts and birthing centres may have their own guidelines for who can access their provisions. This might mean that anyone with a BMI of over 35 is automatically classed as 'high risk', and therefore the option of home birth is presumed to be unavailable. Unlike access to a birthing centre or water birth, the option to birth at home cannot be gatekept or removed from some service users based on BMI. In fact, HCPs have a duty of care to attend you in labour; although this duty of care might be mitigated by sending paramedics to you in labour, you should not be told, or made to feel, that you are not allowed to give birth at home.

Your HCP is required by their code of conduct to provide you with the information that you need to make an informed decision. This doesn't have to be the same decision that they would come to, either professionally or personally. It also doesn't mean that you are required to continue a conversation once you have made your decision. For example, I was at an appointment with a doula client once who said, very plainly, 'I do not want to be induced; I decline induction.' After a bit of back and forth, the HCP said that she was required to listen to him talk about the risks of not having induction. This is unfortunately a fairly common misinterpretation of an important legal case that set the precedent for informed consent and sharing of information: *Montgomery v. Lanarkshire Health Board* (2015).

Montgomery v. Lanarkshire clarified the law on what is required of a healthcare professional when discussing the risks and benefits of any aspect of medical care. Mrs Montgomery sued the Lanarkshire health board after her baby was injured during his birth, stating that she had not been given enough information to make an informed decision about her birth options. The court agreed and the judgment explained that patients have the right to be given all of the information that would be relevant and important to them as an individual. The Montgomery case can sometimes be misinterpreted by midwives and doctors to mean that they are also obligated to tell a pregnant women or person about all the risks and benefits of *not* accepting an intervention, test, medication etc. This is not quite true. 'They are obligated to offer to tell you, you are not obliged to listen.'[3]

You are also not required to sign any waivers relating to your choices. You may be asked to sign something to (paraphrasing here) absolve the hospital/trust/professionals of any possible litigation based on your choices. For example, I was asked to sign a 'women's choice' document as I was birthing at home against medical advice.

To sign to decline treatment or intervention makes no sense when you consider the starting point of healthcare. The professional code of conduct, the laws and regulations surrounding healthcare – these all function on the centralization of informed consent and patient-centred care. Even if it's phrased as 'To have a home birth you need to sign a waiver', you don't. This would be an example of coerced consent.

If consent is sought for certain treatments, medications etc., and to get consent they use false or misleading information ('You can't have a home birth because of your BMI'), threat ('If you choose to birth at home you have to sign away your rights; we will refer you to social services etc.') or fear of what will happen if you don't consent ('If you birth at home your baby will die'), this is coerced consent. If you don't have the option of saying 'no', then any consent given is coerced.

The NHS Constitution for England confirms:

You have the right to be treated with dignity and respect, in

---

3   https://shop.aims.org.uk/products/aims-guide-to-your-rights-in-pregnancy-birth, p.39.

accordance with your human rights. You have the right to accept or refuse treatment that is offered to you, and not to be given any physical examination or treatment unless you have given valid consent. If you do not have the capacity to do so, consent must be obtained from a person legally able to act on your behalf, or the treatment must be in your best interests. You have the right to be given information about the test and treatment options available to you, what they involve and their risks and benefits.[4]

Or, as Emma Ashworth, AIMS trustee and author of *The AIMS Guide to Your Rights in Pregnancy and Birth*, puts it:

Every doctor, every midwife, every healthcare provider involved in your care, whether you're having a straightforward pregnancy or one with many complications, is obliged both by law and their own code of conduct to recognize that the only person who can make decisions about your body is you. If a midwife or doctor is offering any form of test or intervention, they are obliged by law to offer to explain what it is, why they are offering it and the risks and benefits of it.[5]

There are many reasons why people choose to give birth at home – from worries over childcare for older children to past experiences of medical trauma. There are no 'acceptable' reasons to want a home birth; there are just your reasons. You are not required to justify or convince your healthcare professionals of your position. They may be curious and want to know if there is anything they can help you with given their expertise and training, but you don't have to convince them that you are allowed to have a home birth – hopefully I've now dispelled that myth.

Home birth is seen very differently across the world, across time and across cultures. All of my mum's eight siblings, including my mum and

---

4 www.gov.uk/government/publications/the-nhs-constitution-for-england/the-nhs-constitution-for-england

5 https://shop.aims.org.uk/products/aims-guide-to-your-rights-in-pregnancy-birth, p.36.

a set of twins, were born at home – at home in rural Northern Ireland from 1940 something to 1960 something. My nan told me once that the midwife came on a push bike – very *Call the Midwife*. Having said that, there is a gap from my generation to our elders or loved ones who had a home birth. Since my aforementioned rural Northern Irish nan, my family would wait 51 years – until Emma was born in 2015 at home into the water – for the next home birth in our lineage. Emma was joined at the 'I was born at home' club by my nephew Bill a few years later. Considering the number of cousins, aunties, elders and weans running about throughout my life, I don't recall any of them being born at home, apart from a family friend having her third son at home when I was about ten in the late 1990s. I am not alone in this gap of home birthing from our grannies to ourselves. This certainly isn't the book where we explore such a topic, no matter how tantalizing I find it. Suffice to say that as a mammalian species it makes sense that we crave home in labour and birth – home comforts, home smells, home food, home love and home safety. There may be added considerations for fat folks in choosing to stay home. Previous experiences of fatphobia, size bias and medical weight stigma may fuel or influence our decision to choose to birth at home. So what does the research, stats or data say about home birth and safety for folks with BMIs over 30 and their babies?

As with other data sets it can be difficult to find your relative risk within large data sets. For example: if the results group all people with a BMI of over 30, this may include some people who have risk factors that other folks with BMIs over 30 do not, such as advanced maternal age, conception history, disabilities or illnesses. Indeed, Oxford University researchers confirmed:

> Among healthy women with straightforward pregnancy, childbirth risks are influenced more by whether someone is a first-time mum than whether they are obese. They found that the chances of first-time mums of normal weight having medical interventions or complications during childbirth are greater than for 'very obese' but otherwise healthy women having a second or subsequent child.[6]

6   www.ox.ac.uk/news/2013-09-11-childbirth-risks-not-same-all-obese-women

This doesn't mean that first-time parents who have decided to have home births are wrong in their choice to birth at home.

Additionally, in 2015 *BJOG: An International Journal of Obstetrics & Gynaecology* published an analysis of the 'Birthplace in England national cohort study' that looked at perinatal and maternal outcomes in planned home and obstetric unit births in women at 'higher risk' of complications, and concluded:

> In 'higher risk' women, compared with planned OU [obstetric unit] birth, planned home birth was associated with a significantly reduced risk of 'intrapartum related mortality and morbidity' or neonatal admission within 48 hours for more than 48 hours. The difference reflected a higher neonatal admission rate in planned OU births... Compared with planned OU birth, planned home birth was associated with a significantly lower risk of intrapartum interventions and adverse maternal outcomes requiring obstetric care in both nulliparous and parous 'higher risk' women and a significantly higher probability of straightforward vaginal birth in both nulliparous and parous 'higher risk' women.[7]

Dr Sara Wickham discussed these findings, and clarified:

> It is uncertain, however, whether the increase in neonatal admissions reflects an actual difference in morbidity or is due to some other reason, for example perhaps healthcare providers are more likely to recommend transferring babies to a neonatal unit 'just in case'. Women and midwives have long been concerned that intervention is more likely in hospital and that this often occurs when it is not really warranted, and this may be reflective of that.[8]

There is no study that conclusively proves that you, in your unique circumstances, time and place, are safer at home or in hospital. You also

---

7   https://pubmed.ncbi.nlm.nih.gov/26334076, p.43.
8   www.sarawickham.com/research-updates/home-birth-also-safer-for-higher-risk-women

don't need to make that decision by x week of your pregnancy. It may be easier to get you referred to the home birth team if you let your healthcare professional know of your intention to birth at home sooner rather than later, but coming to that decision at a later time than most doesn't prohibit you from having a home birth. Likewise, renting doesn't inhibit your ability to home birth. Neither does not having a show home. As long as there is enough room for your pool (if you are having one), space for midwives (if you are having them attend) to move around you and a flat surface for baby, if needed, you are grand.

Home birth also gets a bad rap in the general cultural sphere. It's draped in misogynistic misconceptions rooted in how unclean and undignified it must be to not have an endless supply of inco (incontinence) pads and freshly laundered sheets. Most home births that I have attended have required less clean up than my dining table when my children have been let loose with the messy craft box. Maybe that says more about my children than home birth. As a rough idea for home birth, here is a generalized list of resources that may make home birth easier, practically speaking.

First, towels! These absolutely do not have to be John Lewis' finest 1000 thread count. In all home births that I have played a part in, a loved one, community member or charity shop has been able to provide what is needed. You also don't need 5000 of them. It's hard to put a firm number on them, especially as size of towels, and people, vary dramatically. To start with, aim to have enough to cover your chosen labouring space. This might be your bedroom, bathroom, front room or the like. You've likely already built up a picture in your mind of where and how you will labour (in a birthing pool, in a pool, on the bed etc.) so plan to have enough to comfortably cover these areas. If you are having a water birth, have a few to cover the surrounding area of the pool as well as to wrap baby and yourself in. If any of your support people are getting in the pool with you, make sure to have a towel for them as well. Add a couple for good measure and any that aren't used can be offered back to the community, charity shops or, if you have a sewing machine, you can fashion reusable baby wipes by cutting squares and top stitching the edges!

One or two sturdy bin bags – not the wafty, hanging-on-by-the-skin-of-their-teeth almost translucent kind. Invest in a couple of proper bags. These can be used for disposing of towels, pads, inco pads, bags of vomit – you name it. The last thing you need a few days after giving birth is the bag ripping on its journey to the kerb.

Waterproof sheets. Found surprisingly affordably in discount stores – sometimes styled as dust sheets or even shower curtains. You could even reuse camping ground sheets or the like. Sitting on this on its own is uncomfortable, so place it under a towel or old sheet that you don't mind being stained or binned.

Other things in my doula bag just make sense: straws, hair ties, eye mask, ear plugs, essential oils/something nice to smell, spare socks, fluffy socks, coconut oil (can be used for massage, dry skin, dry lips and so much more), snacks, (new) toothbrush and toothpaste, headphones, power bank, torch, flannel/wash cloth, and more snacks.

If you are using a birth pool, the first consideration is your boiler. Combi or water heater? This is going to impact your ability to quickly fill the pool. However, even if you have a small hot water heater, this doesn't mean that a home water birth is off the table. Once my hot water heater had been emptied during Emma's birth my doula set about filling pots and heating them on the stove. Another way to mitigate a small or time-sensitive filling of the birth pool is to use a smaller one. Some pools are bigger than others and allow for more than one person to be comfortable in the pool for longer periods. The other consideration with a birth pool is how you fill and drain it. Every house has different set-ups, and finding an adapter to match your nearest tap can be tricky. The best thing to do is to go to your nearest hardware store with a photo of your taps. If you are really struggling, you can use one of several hacks, like the cola bottle hack (attaching the hose to the neck of the cola bottle and cutting a hole in the side to slide it over the tap), or siphoning the water from a (clean) sink into the pool. When deciding where to put the pool it can be useful to consider where the nearest drain/sink/toilet is to drain the water into. If you have access to outdoor space, remember to check outside in the garden – there could be a drain that is closer outside.

Another thing that might help your plans for home birth run smoothly is preparing your boundaries for others' opinions on your choices. There is no shortage of people whose experiences, or the experiences of their loved ones, means that they would never choose home birth. One of my nearest and dearest, Helen, had almost the exact opposite opinion of home birth than I did. She felt it too prehistoric, too risky and too messy. I considered my giving birth to Emma at hospital to be too modern, too risky and too messy...emotionally. Emma, and Helen's second child, were born six weeks apart (our eldest ten weeks apart too), and we had many conversations surrounding our birth plans throughout our pregnancies – especially as this usually meant watching our two-and-a-half-year-olds run around and tire themselves out while we sat with drinks and snacks. We were able to navigate a difference in our realities in very similar circumstances. Our age, ethnicity, parous, both with a BMI of over 30, conception method, background and geographical location were as close to similar as can be, yet we both arrived at different decisions that felt right for us. Unfortunately, not everyone is lucky enough to have a Helen in their lives, and you may find people have very strong opinions on your choosing home birth. 'Especially at your...size.'

Feel free to dispatch the faux-concerned folks in whatever method feels most comfortable to you. Be that 'You aren't a part of my birth team or healthcare team so don't discuss my body, my choices or my baby – cheers' to 'I appreciate your concern, but I have arrived at my decision, and I am not looking for any more information or input into those decisions right now.' You do not have to allow others free space to step on you.

I appreciate that this is harder said than done in a culture that has allowed others to comment on, or indeed touch, pregnant people's bodies and to comment on their birth choices with near impunity for so long. If you are not the gestational parent, but you do love the gestational parent and want to know about their birth plans so that you can help and provide loving support, rather than asking, 'You're having it in hospital, right?' perhaps try, 'If you are comfortable, I would love to hear all about your birth plans! We're really excited to be able to help if there is anything we can support you with.'

CHAPTER 12

Induction of Labour

There are plenty of books, blogs and podcasts dedicated to the subject of induction of labour and I do not presume to know more than those. I will, however, remind you of a theme that is hopefully emerging by now: me proposing a title or discussion point, and then immediately reminding you, dear reader, that it is your choice.

So it will come as no surprise that again, first and foremost, accepting an offer of induction is optional. 'But...but...but...' I hear you call!

Regardless of anything, as we covered previously with our discussion on *Am I Allowed? What Every Woman Should Know BEFORE She Gives Birth* (Beverley Ann Lawrence Beech, 2014) and *The AIMS Guide to Your Rights in Pregnancy and Birth*,[1] all interventions and treatment offers are optional. Including induction.

Many women and birthing people find induction of labour to be a positive experience. There are also folks who may find reassurance in the extra monitoring while awaiting spontaneous labour; if this isn't offered, do ask your healthcare provider about expectant management options. As with all offers of intervention there is no right answer as to whether you should accept or decline these offers.

A common justification for induction of labour is going 'overdue' or 'post-dates'. Forty weeks from the date of your last period is used to calculate your due date. This is seldom baby's birthday, and, like wizards, babies are neither late, nor early; they arrive precisely when they mean to. In the global north we are often obsessed with due

---

1   https://shop.aims.org.uk/products/aims-guide-to-your-rights-in-pregnancy-birth

dates, even though only 5 per cent of babies arrive on their due date.[2] Because of the framing of due dates as an expiration date rather than a general estimation of window of arrival, many parents understandably consider 40 weeks + 1 day pregnant to be overdue. However, 'term' means 37–42 weeks. Therefore, you technically aren't 'post-dates' or 'overdue' until 42 + 1.

Here is some of the data on unexplained stillbirth at various gestations from *Inducing Labour* by Dr Sara Wickham:[3]

- 35 weeks: 1 in 500
- 36 weeks: 1 in 556
- 37 weeks: 1 in 645
- 38 weeks: 1 in 730
- 39 weeks: 1 in 840
- 40 weeks: 1 in 926
- 41 weeks: 1 in 826
- 42 weeks: 1 in 769
- 43 weeks: 1 in 633.

It's worth pointing out that using this data set it can be argued that giving birth at 43 weeks is more or less as likely to end in an unexplained stillbirth than giving birth during week 37 of pregnancy: 1 in 633 compared to 1 in 645. Or indeed, comparing 42 weeks at 1 in 769 to 1 in 730 at 38 weeks.

More and more people are having their labours induced: 'According to NHS Maternity Statistics, the proportion of labours in England that are induced has increased from 21% in the year to March 2010 to 34% in the year to March 2021.'[4] More than a third of people giving birth in the UK had their labours induced! That is a remarkable statistic, whichever way you slice it.

Agreeing to an induction will limit your birth choices and plans to some extent. It is likely that you will be asked to consent to repeated

---

2   https://pubmed.ncbi.nlm.nih.gov/23932061
3   www.sarawickham.com/iol, p.74.
4   www.aims.org.uk/journal/item/induction-birth-information

vaginal examinations to assess your dilation and effacement, as well as being required to be on the labour ward (rather than the birthing suite or at home) to be induced. Depending on your local hospital or trust's guidelines, this might mean being alone for part of this process overnight or outside of visiting hours and continuous monitoring – likely by sensors placed onto your belly that track baby's heartbeat as well as measure contractions – with large elastic bands looped around your belly to hold them in place. This can limit your freedom of movement (the sensors can shift during movement and make it harder to get a reading of baby's heart rate). It will also likely restrict your use of water (although some hospitals have waterproof wireless monitors – which, when working and not currently in use, should enable continuous monitoring without the wires). It is also often reported that induced labours are more painful than spontaneous labours because they are being augmented chemically. Other risks include hyperstimulation (the uterus contracts too frequently, or contractions last too long, which can lead to changes in foetal heart rate and result in foetal compromise), higher likelihood of instrumental delivery (and the complications associated with instrumental delivery such as perineal and sphincter injuries and tears), as well as a higher likelihood of unplanned caesarean birth and longer hospital admissions.[5]

The sprint audit[6] on BMI and pregnancy concluded: 'Further research is required to determine the optimum gestation of induction, to improve the accuracy of antenatal diagnosis, and to determine whether induction of labour is also beneficial in women with a BMI of 30 kg/m^2 or above.'

Before induction of labour on the labour ward you may be offered something called a 'membrane sweep', 'stretch and sweep', or sometimes just a 'sweep'. This is where your healthcare provider (usually a doctor or midwife) carries out a vaginal examination and then uses their finger in a sweeping motion around the inside of your cervix.

---

5   www.nice.org.uk/guidance/ng207/chapter/Recommendations
6   https://maternityaudit.org.uk/FilesUploaded/NMPA%20BMI%20Over%2030%20Report.pdf, p.9.

NICE recommends[7] that a sweep is offered at an antenatal appointment after 39 weeks, with a subsequent sweep offered if labour does not start spontaneously following the first sweep.

A Cochrane Review[8] on sweeps showed that there may be little or no difference between groups (those who had a sweep and those who didn't) regarding the likelihood of having an unplanned caesarean, spontaneous vaginal birth, maternal death or serious morbidity, and neonatal perinatal death or serious morbidity. It did state, however, that 'women randomised to membrane sweeping may be more likely to experience spontaneous onset of labour (low-certainty evidence) but less likely to experience induction.'

The Review concluded: 'Membrane sweeping may be effective in achieving a spontaneous onset of labour, but the evidence for this was of low certainty. When compared to expectant management, it potentially reduces the incidence of formal induction of labour. Questions remain as to whether there is an optimal number of membrane sweeps and timings and gestation of these to facilitate induction of labour.'[9]

Various methods of induction may be used depending on the hospital and your unique circumstances. Cervical ripening may be the first stage of the induction process. Being offered synthetic prostaglandin pessaries, gel or a tablet inserted into the vagina is a common method of induction of labour. For some people this is 'enough' or a kick-start that the body required, and labour can continue as 'normal' from this point. However, if cervical ripening is not 'enough', the HCP may then offer to break your waters – if your cervix has ripped enough to allow access to an implement, not entirely non-crochet-hook-like, inserted through the cervix to rupture the amniotic sac. It is also possible that you may be offered catheter or balloon cervical ripening methods rather than chemical ripening. This is sometimes called manual cervix ripening whereas the previous methods are chemical

---

7   www.nice.org.uk/guidance/ng207/chapter/Recommendations#methods-for-induction-of-labour
8   www.cochranelibrary.com/cdsr/doi/10.1002/14651858.CD000451.pub3/full, p.2.
9   www.cochranelibrary.com/cdsr/doi/10.1002/14651858.CD000451.pub3/full, p.3.

ripening. Manual cervical ripening does exactly what is says on the tin. It uses a Foley balloon or catheter to apply gentle pressure to the cervix to encourage it to open. Once the cervix is dilated enough to allow a practitioner to feel the sac, they can artificially rupture membranes (ARM) or manually break your waters.

Like other methods of labour induction, ARM has a number of downsides:

- It can speed up contractions and, while this can help to progress labour, some women find this easier to cope with than others.
- It can cause pain to increase faster than when women are in spontaneous labour.
- It carries an increased chance of infection.
- There is a chance of umbilical cord prolapse (where the cord slips in front of the baby's head, necessitating an immediate crash caesarean), although this is rare. It can cause the baby not to cope as well with labour as it would have done had the onset of labour been spontaneous.

One other important thing to know is that once a woman's waters have released, either naturally or by artificial means, caregivers tend to take the position that everyone is now committed to the continuation of the induction, since the risk of infection to the baby is increased by breaking the foetal membranes.[10]

Guidelines on induction of labour or baby to be born via caesarean section after spontaneous rupture of waters vary across trusts and hospitals, from 24–72 hours, due to risk of infection. When deciding if you would like to accept your providers' offer of induction it might be another time to use your BRAIN: Benefits, Risks, Alternatives, Intuition, Nothing (see Chapter 7).

---

10   www.sarawickham.com/iol, p.27.

An interview with Kate from Lesbemums

To hear more about mothers' and gestational parents' stories of induction I spoke to my mate Kate. I met Kate online through her LGBTQ+ parenting and lifestyle account Lesbemums. Kate is a lesbian mum who works in the public sector. She lives in Brighton with her wife Sharon and their son, who is eight.

*

AJ: Induction is such a varied process, and how induction is experienced by parents varies so hugely I just don't think that we can hear too many stories about this process for hopeful or expectant parents to hear about induction.

Kate: So, I was two weeks over, they didn't want to do an induction until I was overdue. For some LGBTQ+ people (and people using assisted conception) it's sometimes slightly different than for people who conceive via penis in vagina sex. We know when we ovulated, and we know when insemination happened. So we had worked out when he would be due ourselves, and by our calculations we were spot on (40 weeks), but the midwife said I was two weeks late.

AJ: Based on their calculations that differed from your own?

Kate: Yes, they calculated basically two weeks extra on top, based on the scan, I think she said, but it was a while ago now! If Sharon was here, she would remember!

AJ: And by two weeks late I imagine she meant 42 weeks rather than 44?

Kate: Yes, it was 42 weeks and a day or two; again, Sharon would know!

AJ: An estimate will do I reckon for the purpose of our conversation...

Kate: I am pretty sure I was 42 weeks and a day or so when I went in for the pessary. She said, 'We will book you in for the drip as well the day after the pessary if it doesn't work.' When I got the pessary, oh my god, I have never been in so much pain, it was worse than giving birth. It was quite an uncomfortable experience inserting it, but for me, it was almost instantaneous! As soon as it was in things really ramped up. When I was chatting with them when I was being observed before I could go home with the pessary, we were saying to them 'things are really ramping up' and the attitude we got back was very much 'not this quickly, we know you are done being pregnant, but you are exaggerating', basically. Then, by the time we could leave the hospital, I could barely walk, but they sent me home and that was pretty much the rest of my labour at home – me in pain and Sharon on the phone to the birthing unit once every couple of hours and them dismissing us. What I wanted was to be in the hospital and have a water birth, but when we called up and said we wanted to come in, they looked at the system and saw I had had the pessary only hours ago and they kept saying, 'It won't have had time to work yet' and things like 'Have a bath' or 'Take paracetamol and have a sleep' – things that were just deeply unhelpful. I really started to struggle emotionally because I thought, they must be right, they are the professionals, and they are saying this is early labour. So, I am *fucked* for later stages and pushing – if I am in this much pain now, in what they are calling early labour, then how am I possibly going to cope with what is to come?! Sharon also didn't know what to do because she was the one on the phone with them and she would say to me, 'What should I do? Should I just say we are coming in even though they have said we shouldn't yet?' It's hard to watch your loved one feel that lost, especially when you are doing that between contractions! That was our introduction to labour and birth, that was the start of him coming into the world, and it was spent not really knowing what to do.

AJ: I am hearing a real theme of not being believed, of not being heard.

Kate: Absolutely, and it did make me wonder, if I had been a member of a different community, if I might have been taken more seriously. Between Sharon having to keep explaining she was not calling for herself each time we called, I do wonder if that did impact how they perceived us and my pain. By about 9.30 Sharon had just had enough and said on the phone to them, 'We are coming in now' and they even said to her then, 'Well, if her waters haven't broken, we will send you home again.' Thankfully my waters did break when I was getting into my mum's car, though! So that was something.

AJ: Ahh, it's always when you pop to the loo through the carpeted hallway or when someone with nice trainers on is standing next to you, in my experience!

Kate: Eventually, when we got to the hospital, and bless Sharon, she did manage to pick the one wheelchair that had to be pulled backwards like a B&Q trolley!

AJ: Oh my god, that is such a queer explanation of that type of push–pull situation.

Kate: Well it's true! She was pulling this trolley and then dragging me behind her, trying to find this one lift that goes to the maternity ward, as all the other lifts don't stop at that floor. When we finally got up there and manoeuvred this wheelchair out of the lift, they told us to go over to triage because I wouldn't be in established labour yet, so not the labour ward, right? I get to the triage and was invited into this room, and as soon as I got onto the little table/bed thing the midwife looks and says, 'Oh you are crowning!' Sharon, for the first time, gets a bit animated and is proclaiming, 'I told you, you should have listened to us!' and I am kind of just sitting there, saying, 'It's alright, it's okay' and I am crowning, you know. I don't know if she was a man, would she have been taken more seriously, or would they have listened to her more, I don't know. Sharon was very upset because the labour we had planned and what we thought the hours before our son was born would look like had just been spent with her having the labour unit on speed dial because I was in so much pain and they wouldn't believe us. What hadn't helped was as we were coming through the unit to this triage room, we saw a ward with only one person in one bed and the other five beds were empty, and we had been asking to come in to be checked all day. By the time we really knew what was happening I gave birth to him in the triage room. The birthing unit is one floor up from where I was so we couldn't get up there in time. I was pretty angry, to be honest, but then moments later I saw my son, which made things slightly better. However, I do wonder if this affected my birth, though. Because I tore quite badly, and suffered for a long time with terrible haemorrhoids where my tear was. All the time I was thinking that maybe if I had been in the hospital earlier and on the birthing unit rather than a kind of cold triage room, maybe it would have been different. I wouldn't have been so anxious, and Sharon would haven't have been so stressed, and maybe we would have been able to cuddle up and get into our little love bundle, and maybe I wouldn't have torn. I didn't want to be at home, because of my anxiety. It's just a shame, I guess.

AJ: I am sorry that happened, Sharon. That sounds so stressful and upsetting. Not the ideal start to labour and birth for sure! Can I ask you about when you were offered an induction? Was this during a midwifery appointment or was it an obstetrician? Did you feel like you were given all the information you needed to make an informed decision?

Kate: It was a midwife, and definitely not. I mean, they told me the pessary was kind of like a tampon that releases a chemical that does this, that and the other. She didn't seem overly convinced it would work, to be honest.

AJ: How so?

Kate: Well, she kept saying things like, 'It doesn't work very often' and, 'We usually end up doing the drip anyway, so I'll book you in for that the day after.' She checked me and checked where he (the baby) was etc., but they were quite nonchalant about it really. Maybe I am in the minority of people who have a strong reaction to the pessary because when he came out, the pessary was stuck to his head!

AJ: I mean, I don't know the stats about how many people go on to labour with 'just' the pessary, but I wonder what impact it has on people when HCPs phrase it like 'It's not going to work', right?

Kate: I asked her why they couldn't just go straight to the drip, then, and she said we must follow the guidelines, basically. I asked another question and I felt like she was getting bit annoyed with me asking questions, and then when Sharon asked another one, we both just felt like we couldn't ask anymore. We felt that we were taking up too much of her time or that she didn't want to answer our questions really. She just kept saying, 'It's a routine thing, don't worry, it will be fine.' Which isn't as reassuring as she thinks it is, I think. I wanted to ask if she thought it wasn't going to work because I was fat, or did she say this to everyone? I felt completely uninformed about why she was saying that it wasn't going to work, and confused about why they had to do it if she was so sure that it wasn't going to work.

AJ: Did she say why you were being offered induction?

Kate: Literally just dates – even though there were no complications in my pregnancy with me or with the baby. I have met someone who refused induction, but I didn't feel confident enough to do that. I don't think I am alone in thinking that you just do what the professionals tell you? You know? They know! Of course, they know! 'You say I should do XYZ, then of course I am going to do it, because you are the professional, you've trained to do this', you know?

AJ: You aren't alone, no, especially in the UK where we don't pay at the point of care for our healthcare. We do pay for our healthcare, of course, just by a different method than getting a bill after you leave.

But I think having this free at the point of contact, and moreover the British kind of 'Don't rock the boat' and the misogynistic 'be a good girl and do as you are told' kind of thing...

Kate: Since talking to other people and hearing their stories I feel as if I should have asked more questions, I should have dug my heels in a bit, I suppose. It was very strange; you just go along with it, especially because you are so excited to meet your baby and you can't wait to hold them and love them, and if they are offering to make that happen sooner, why not!

AJ: Oh 100 per cent, a lot of people feel similarly and don't realize that you can decline their offers of induction, or any other intervention that they offer. They don't usually make it sound like an offer, though, so I understand why it happens.

Kate: Yes, it was very much 'We'll do this, then we'll do that', without a break or a pause in between for discussion.

AJ: Sounds a lot like not being heard or listened to again, sounds familiar, right?

Kate: Yes, throughout the pregnancy it felt very nurtured and easy. The midwife telling you 'Make sure you rest' and all this lovely stuff, and then as soon as we got to the induction it just felt rushed. It felt like they couldn't process you through fast enough and they wanted you out the door as soon as possible. I appreciate that it seems like pregnant folks are more delicate in the early stages, but even at 42 weeks I still felt delicate and vulnerable. I needed to be held and comforted, and the induction process just didn't feel like that at all. It was strange to go from calm, loving and nurturing care to 'Let's just get the baby out asap.'

AJ: Thinking about your wider care, were there any other aspects of your care, including conception care, that you felt were impacted because of your size?

Kate: I think certainly in the early stages when people were finding out that he was donor conceived they were very keen in finding out about the donor. I'm not completely ignorant in why they need to know; they need to find out if there are any genetic conditions that we need to be aware of and the like. But they were completely consumed with finding out his BMI. One person did call him 'dad'; thankfully they quickly corrected themselves, but they were so consumed with his BMI. Then, when we said, 'Well, we don't know too much but we do know his rough size from his description', and I could see them looking at me, and almost calculating on the spot if fat + fat would cause any issues. While I do appreciate that they have to ask some of these questions, I do think that they could have handled it more sensitively. Sometimes I didn't know if it was a necessary question, you know?

AJ: Mmmm, yes, as LGBTQ+ people we are used to a different level of inappropriate curiosity and the dreaded 'Can I ask you...?' once they find out you are queer!

Kate: I didn't know where the line was, you know? I didn't have any family to help advise me or guide me through what would usually be asked at appointments, or anyone to come with me who had been through this before who would know that a question was out of place. I just always answered the questions, even in situations where I felt uncomfortable. I didn't want to be argumentative.

AJ: Inappropriate curiosity is a big problem for LGBTQ+ people (48% of LGBTQ people have experienced this"), and particularly in pregnancy because there is so much misinformation and so much is unknown!

---

11   https://blogs.bmj.com/bmj/2019/09/09/trans-health-and-the-risks-of-inappropriate-curiosity

There is a clear line, however, between inappropriate curiosity and 'I need to know this to do my job, i.e., was your baby donor conceived?' This makes a difference to the care pathway, right? But just because you need to ask people that question doesn't mean that you can just blurt it out in whatever way you want. Another example is, if you've got a two-mum family in front of you and you need to ask who the gestational mother is because you are about to help them with infant feeding, that is going to impact the lactation advice and information you give to them. Just because you need to know the answer to that question doesn't mean that you can say, 'Who's the real mum?'!

Kate: Erg! Yes!

AJ: Asking the question and giving justification like 'Can I ask who the gestational mother is because that will change my advice based on inducing lactation or spontaneous lactation' takes an extra 10 seconds and reassures us that you are aware that we are used to being asked all kinds of inappropriate and invasive questions.

Kate: I do think some explanation would have been helpful and reassuring that it wasn't just because we were a two-mum family. You also want to be like a 'good gay' or a 'good fat mum'. There are a lot of things that looking back now I would do differently, I think.

AJ: What would you do differently?

Kate: I think I wouldn't be as worried about asking, 'Why do you need to know that?' or, 'Would you ask me that if I wasn't fat or if I was married to a man?' etc. Obviously, there are some extra questions that you expect to answer being part of a slightly, I guess, 'unusual' family. But I do think that there was a kind of 'give them an inch and they will take a mile' happening with the questioning. Even when I was at home and I was learning to breastfeed they would say things that just didn't make sense for me and my body. The first time someone came round to help us with feeding, Sharon was holding the baby and I answered the door and when she came into the living room she started chatting to Sharon and she said to her, 'Let's have a look then' and Sharon handed the baby to me, and the midwife just didn't know what to do! I think because Sharon is a fat woman, too, that increases the chances of people mistaking her for the gestational mother, but again, it felt like they were just trying to use the same old advice and information that they give to the majority of parents.

AJ: Who aren't fat and who likely are a heterosexual couple.

Kate: Absolutely. There was just this assumption that she was the gestational mother or that she was the parent who was feeding the baby because she was the one holding the baby and I was the one who got up and answered the door.

AJ: Ah, the answer is patriarchy and misogyny again! The gestational mum must be the one caring for the baby because non-gestational parents or fathers don't do that!

Kate: Yeah, that is bullshit! Even when Sharon passed the baby over, the midwife said, 'Ah, giving mum a break.' Sharon just said, 'I'm going to go and make tea.' I think it was only because then I had my boobs out and my newborn baby on me that I felt quite vulnerable. You think, if I say something or question the information that I am being given, are you going to react badly? Are you going to withhold care or not give me as much time as the other people who didn't question you? So when you already feel vulnerable it feels impossible to put yourself out there and risk compromising your care. Just be quiet and don't rock the boat. Be a good mum or a good gay.

AJ: Is there anything that you would want to tell fat people about induction or about wider fat pregnancy experiences?

Kate: I wish I had asked, 'Do I have to do this or are there any other options?' more often. From being weighed or discussing my BMI at every appointment to induction. Speak to other fat parents and other people who have had similar experiences. I think a lot of people are scared because they say things like, 'This baby has to come out' and, 'What is the risk if we wait, or if we do something else?' Speak to other parents who live near you as well and seek out informed or inclusive providers. Most of all, don't be afraid to advocate for yourself.

AJ: If you could speak to the providers, then, what would you say about fat people and induction to them?

Kate: I guess it is very 'every day' at work for you, but for us this is not something we've ever experienced before, and so this doesn't happen every day to us. It's brand new, it's scary, we feel and we are very vulnerable. We need love. We need reassurance. Please listen to us! Just because we have loads of fat doesn't mean that we can't feel that we are contracting! It doesn't mean that we are stupid or that we don't know what we are talking about! Things might happen outside of the average or outside of the norm that the statistics say they will, and please listen to us if that happens. Even if you think that we are just panicking, reassure us; don't dismiss us.

AJ: Such wise words, my darling, thank you. I am also asking everyone about their favourite fat pregnancy consumable. Whether that's a brand of maternity wear that has inclusive sizing or a product like a feeding pillow, or whatever is good for fat folks. Do you have anything that you would recommend to hopeful or expectant fat parents?

Kate: Oh, I loved, when I was pumping, when I went back to work, my pump, because it had really big, erm, caps or whatever they are called, for big nipples!

AJ: Flange! I love that word!

Kate: Yes, thank you, flange! It was a Lansinoh® manual pump, and it came with various sizes, and those were the biggest ones I could find. The other ones I tried were tiny. I was spilling out of them and then the air seal would get broken, or it was compressing my nipple and rubbing up against the side and it would be really painful. I had massive boobs before pregnancy anyway, but when I was feeding, they kept growing and growing, so having a pump that came with different-sized, and larger-sized, flanges was important. Oh, and the baby sling! We struggled because Sharon is very broad, and I have a large chest so between us we really needed two different carriers, because what would work for her shoulders would be too tight around the chest for me. It wasn't until we went to the local sling library, and they helped us with a long fabric sling instead, that we found a sling that we could both use. The buckled ones with all the big bits of padding were just never going to work for me or for Sharon. They just aren't made for people of our size.

AJ: No, they aren't. These firms have an idea of their target or average market, and we aren't that. We aren't in any of the pictures, or in the minds of the people when they make it, so why would it fit us?

Kate: Depressing, but true.

AJ: Is there anything else that we haven't covered or spoken about that you think that parents need to hear?

Kate: I would definitely say that being fat isn't an indicator of how fertile you are. When we were struggling to conceive, I would always be sitting there thinking it's because I am so fat, it's because I am fat. And even the people you would go to for help would say, 'It's because of your size.' Slim people have fertility issues, too, so beating yourself up or convincing yourself that it is because you are fat doesn't help. You should be given equal opportunities and rights to access fertility services. Your body size doesn't change your worth.

*

Kate's experience is far from individual, and fat folks often exist at an intersection of identities. We may be fat at the same time as being LGBTQ, disabled, racialized, impoverished or unhoused. The ways our individual identities, circumstances and lives intersect with our fatness will change the way the people and the systems perceive us. Often, we are perceived as less than – less worthy of time, consideration, help or love. So remember Kate's wise words: *Your body size doesn't change your worth.*

CHAPTER 13

Perinatal and Fat

Lactation, slings and carriers

Having been a fat breastfeeding parent I have heard, first hand, many of the common tropes regarding BMI and lactation. Whether that takes shape as tropes about breast size and lactation success rates, or that fat parents are less likely to feed because of their restrictions in movement. I've heard them all. Don't just take my word for it.

Looking at the results from a survey on the relationship between maternal BMI with the onset of breastfeeding from the *International Breastfeeding Journal* studies[1] they get tantalizingly close to identifying the difficulties. This study identifies that mothers with a raised BMI are less likely to have skin to skin with their infants in the first hour after birth. We also know that 'a quarter more women who have this contact with their babies are still breastfeeding at one to four months after birth compared with those who don't'.[2] We know that folks with a higher BMI are more likely to experience induction of labours, caesarean births, and emergency caesarean birth.[3] We know about the existing relationship between caesarean section[4] and a disparity in initiation of breastfeeding[5] as well as induction of labour and

---

1   https://internationalbreastfeedingjournal.biomedcentral.com/articles/10.1186/ s13006-020-00298-5
2   https://evidence.nihr.ac.uk/alert/skin-to-skin-contact-improves-breastfeeding-of-healthy-babies
3   https://obgyn.onlinelibrary.wiley.com/doi/pdf/10.1111/aogs.12263
4   www.unicef.org.uk/babyfriendly/impact-of-labour-interventions
5   https://bmcpregnancychildbirth.biomedcentral.com/articles/10.1186/s12884-020-2732-6

lactation.[6] Karin Cadwell's 2018 speakers' series for UNICEF concluded, 'No positive relationships between the administration of synthetic oxytocin and breastfeeding were found.'[7]

So this all begs the question: is the medicalization of fat birth causing or even contributing to the disparities of breastfeeding initiation rates in fat folks? Add on top of this the disparities of access of feeding supplies (bras, pump flanges) as well as a lack of fat-friendly resources and of fat-inclusive training in professionals supporting lactation. That's all before we even touch on how fat women's bodies are more likely to be expected to be hidden and covered in a society and culture that already doesn't support public feeding – is it any wonder that fat folks aren't being supported to feed? I asked Emma Pickett, IBCLC (International Board of Certified Lactation Consultant), former chair of the Association of Breastfeeding Mothers, author of three books on the subject of lactation and breasts (Warning: it is possible that your ten-year-old child will help themselves to *The Breast Book* from your office shelf, read it cover to cover, and then come to you, a birth and postnatal doula, breastfeeding councillor, a parent who breastfed their two children for over seven years combined, and teach you about breastfeeding. It's wonderful - highly recommended), and all-round lactation oracle, what her thoughts were on the above:

> The most significant barrier to bigger parents breastfeeding successfully is not their own body but society's attitude to their body. In nearly two decades of supporting families, I can count on one hand the videos I have seen showing a fat person breastfeeding or chest-feeding. Every day assumptions are made about standard positions and breast and nipple shapes that don't fit everyone and leave parents feeling abandoned and isolated. Descriptions are given that expect a straight size or thin body and a front facing nipple. Despite an explosion of resources via the internet, the situation is still dire. Fat inclusive resources and messages are desperately needed.

6   www.unicef.org.uk/babyfriendly/impact-of-labour-interventions
7   www.unicef.org.uk/babyfriendly/impact-of-labour-interventions/?sisearchengi ne=1022

Interview with Vanisha Virgo

Thinking about my lived experience as a fat postnatal parent and my professional experience being a doula for fat folks, I was continually reminded that fat folks aren't expected to be here. We aren't the default imagery of happy new motherhood. That thought led me to Vanisha Virgo, a birth and postnatal doula I have been lucky enough to train and work alongside many times. Watching her work for improving access for Black mothers, I knew there was no one better to have this conversation with than Vanisha.

*

AJ: First, it's got to be said. We've had this conversation many times. Conversations that haven't been planned and haven't been recorded, but here we are now, doing it for real! So, knowing we were coming together today to have the recorded interview for the book, what has been on your mind leading up to today?

Vanisha: It's ignorance! Stop being ignorant. Fat isn't unhealthy. Fat is sexy, fat is juicy, fat is delicious. Fat isn't an illness. Just because I have a voluptuous figure and massive ta tas doesn't mean I am unhealthy. It doesn't mean I am sick. Stop assuming I am sitting down, shoving food in my face watching Netflix all day because I am fat.

AJ: I mean, I do that. I do sit and watch Netflix and eat food! Right? But that doesn't remove from me the basic and universal right to humanity and dignity, right?

Vanisha: Exactly. And, err, hello? Fat and muscle can look the same under clothing. BMI is bullshit. Can we stop with that shit please? Shove it up your arse. I'm done being kind and gentle about it; they aren't kind or gentle with it to me.

AJ: Our discussion is going to focus on the perinatal care side of things. Your expertise and experience in this world is huge, and I want to make sure we get as much of your knowledge and wisdom down as possible regarding perinatal care and experiences. Your experience in infant feeding and slings and carriers is going to be unrivalled regarding fat folks. So, first, what are restrictions and difficulties in access that fat folks could experience in perinatal care?

Vanisha: First of, we all know when you are feeding your tiny human or humans you might need some...scaffolding. You need something that is comfortable; my god, I don't want to wear something that looks like my grandma wore when she was pregnant. I want and deserve to feel sexy and comfortable. The restriction in sizing means I know people who only have two bras. Not only because they are hard to find in bigger sizes, but also because they are so expensive. I am an M and not everyone who has a large chest wants to have a reduction, or it's not safe for them to do so. Finding clothing that fits is hard.

AJ: The clothing discussion has come up with everyone I have spoken to. I think it's often batted away as this non-issue, or people think that is the extent of size exclusion or fat bias.

Vanisha: I didn't plan to feed – I went in with bottles – but from my hospital bed I had to order feeding-friendly nightwear. It was January as well, so it was cold and I really needed something to keep me warm and comfortable that I could feed in. I ended up having to go on Amazon and get these Victorian-looking, beige-coloured nightshirts. That was the only thing that I could feed in that was available in my size. I still have them because I was so worried about never finding anything better, and six years later, I haven't found fashionable, comfortable nightwear. I am a hot person, I run hot. Even when I was a skinny person, fat or not, I ran hot. So I don't want thick, like, jumpsuit-type things because I would be sweating and uncomfortable. It must be practical and comfortable. It doesn't have to be fashionable, always, but I deserve to feel good about myself while wearing clothes that are restricted because of how I am using my body, right? What about going out, or to a wedding? It's so difficult to find plus size clothing that is dressy. Especially when I look for natural fibres or materials that breathe better and feel organic next to my skin – it's practically impossible.

AJ: Oh, I run hot, too, we know this from working together, we are both always hot! But if I wear polyester – forget about it! I am 10 degrees cooler in cotton or bamboo than I am in polyester.

Vanisha: I don't wear coats unless it is minus! Even when I was a size 12. But if I am warm and I am feeding my baby, wearing my baby or co-sleeping – that's not good.

AJ: Practicalities aside, what about the restrictions or assumptions that fat people face in perinatal care, then?

Vanisha: I've seen so many in the circles and groups that I run, whether it's slings or feeding groups. In babywearing groups there are posts all the time from the professionals asking, 'I have a client who is a size 20 and they want to know if this carrier fits.' I think to myself, how are you running a sling library or working as a professional in this space if you don't know what size a sling fits up to? They aren't taught this at training. They might talk about petite people and what slings work better for narrow-framed folks, they might also brush up against the topic of big boobs or wider shoulders, but why aren't we sitting down when a new sling or carrier comes out and examining who this might work well for? Who might this not be suitable for? Whether that is regarding disability – the clips on this carrier require two hands to undo, for example. Or this carrier has a stiff waist band, so might put pressure on caesarean birth scars. Why do we leave fat people out of those considerations? We know the minimum and maximum weights for the babies being worn in these slings – why aren't we talking about the maximum or minimum waist size for the wearer?

AJ: That is such a good point. I have done a babywearing consultant course. Granted, it was a long time ago, but I never saw, on any firm's instruction manuals or any press-like leaflets etc., any fat people wearing slings.

Vanisha: That is something I am working towards, inclusive imagery for slings and carriers.

AJ: Yeah, sort 'em out, V! Because you can't be what you can't see, right? So when we are giving out our expertise at the sling library or one-to-one appointments etc., and we are using the language of 'The sling should sit at the smallest part of your waist' or 'Make sure it's not too high up across your back', we are using markers and trying to make it look like how it fits on straight-sized bodies!

Vanisha: Yes!

AJ: So positioning in slings looks very different for straight-sized folks with small breasts than it does for fat people with big boobs.

Vanisha: Exactly. It doesn't consider the belly. For people who are self-conscious of their bellies, they may put on a sling or carrier and see that the carrier's shape is different on them compared to the straight-size imagery in the booklets, and conclude that this carrier isn't suitable or safe for them. It adds to our feelings of not belonging, that babywearing isn't for us because no one in all these images is fat. The world is a nasty place; we don't need to be adding barriers and more harm to folks.

AJ: And most people in this arena, like babywearing consultants and peer supporters, they'll all agree that babywearing is wonderful, even pointing out that this is the norm. As a mammalian species we are hardwired for clinging young – our babies expect to be held or carried. Slings are given out in baby boxes across the world, even in the UK, with Scotland giving out stretchy wraps in their baby boxes too. So why is it, then, in an industry where most, if not all, the professionals will be enamoured to tell you the benefits and the evolutionary backstory, we don't consider knowing what size a carrier goes up to for the wearer important?

Vanisha: Exactly. You can't be what you don't see. And I am going to say it: babywearing is so whitewashed.

AJ: I went to a babywearing expo with Mars Lord, and she pointed this out to a room of stunned and silent attendees. She went round to all the stalls and the concession stands, gathered up their leaflets and took pictures on her phone of their banners, and showed them just how whitewashed this event was.

Vanisha: The thing that gets me is that the babywearing industry, worldwide, is extremely white-centric. Appropriation is key; it is not just common, it is key. I wrote my own course, babywearing training. I won't call it a peer supporter course or consultancy because I am not using the white-centric naming. I included Indigenous cultures from across the world. I learned so much just doing research for that course. There are certain fabrics, ties and colours that have different meanings. And it's never talked about. When people are using history, knowledge and symbols from your culture, repackaging it, and selling it, it's appropriation.

AJ: A common rebuttal is that all societies and cultures carried their young. Like before prams – what did we do? In the course work I did for my consultancy course I found out about my family's history of slings and carriers. I found out about Welsh shawls and how my maternal grandmother used them. She couldn't afford a pram in rural Ireland in the 40s. Plus the roads and terrain weren't suited to prams. The work she had to undertake in rural Ireland in the 40s and 50s when she first became a mother meant she was out in the muddy fields – no all-terrain prams in rural Ireland in 1940, eh? My mum told me it wasn't until my nan had her third child that someone gave her a pram, from her local community. Irish culture means that the descendants of these kind people, who my family still knows, are still, to this day, named as my uncles and aunties. So it isn't that all carrying is appropriative, right? It's that certain carriers, certain colours, patterns and the like are being repackaged in whiteness to make money.

Vanisha: Right. With no mention or discussion of the origins or the history. That, to me, is rage worthy. I had to step away quite a lot because of the refusal to even acknowledge the origins of these carriers. When we look at the experience of Black and Brown folks who want to babywear or to feed their babies, it is problematic to exclude us. Slings and carriers aren't made for fat people. I can't think of a single brand that specifically uses Black and/or fat people in their imagery. You can't be what you can't see.

How do we change that? We must change that from top to toe. We can't just start using more Black and Brown and/or fat models; we need to change the entire system. We need to look at the training, we need to look at the imagery, we need to look at the language, we need to look at the history.

Similarly with breastfeeding. Looking at the imagery used in these courses, for example, mastitis – how that can look on the skin, the pink, red or mottled skin. I've never seen a Black person used in these textbooks or online training resources. Even how to hand express – it's small and pert boobs in the pictures with one-hand expressing happening. I have never, in my entire life, been able to express with one hand; it doesn't work for me. Yet this is the information being given to people who are training to help us?

AJ: One of the things that annoys me is how they show perfectly circular breasts and centralized small nipples. Who is this? I point more at 4pm and 7pm rather than centralized! That changes the whole game regarding positioning and attachment.

Vanisha: All the imagery, all the pictures, all the animations show this. Where my baby has to be, relative to my body, is wildly different to these slides or resources. My nipples point to my elbow, basically, and if I put my baby where they are showing me to put my baby, they are 6 inches from my nipple. We don't talk about these things!

AJ: We don't, again, because of the pursuit of the ideal body; if you fall outside of that ideal, then it must be shameful. We've naturally moved on to talking about breastfeeding, but before we leave slings and carriers to discuss feeding, I want to ask what carriers you recommend for fat folks?

Vanisha: Everyone is different, and fat folks wear their fat in different places, so I don't have a 'top slings for fat people' list. Saying that, there are some things to discuss with fat folks, or that people with large breasts and chests need to know. First, be aware your boobs might be outside of the sling. In the picture I know it's all neat and nothing is hanging out, but that person is a size 10 and we are not all size 10s. Your baby being central on your chest, and the carrier holding them, might mean that your breast or chest is spread wider and therefore comes out the side. That is normal and that is fine. If you don't like that, then get a ring sling.

AJ: I love a ring sling! From memory as well, I mean, I haven't run a sling library in several years, so feel free to jump in and correct me, but I think a Close Caboo is only really going to go up to a size 26. Obviously, dependent on your own shape and size, but it's fixed at a certain length and after that, it isn't going to work.

Vanisha: And it depends on if it's brand new or the material type. Some are stretchier than others.

AJ: I also found that any carrier with thin webbing straps was uncomfortable. The natural valleys and peaks of my body, my rolls, eat up them thin straps, then they dig in and hurt. It also means that my back rolls push the webbing around and then means it's not in a comfortable position. So I personally prefer thicker webbing and more structured carriers because it stays in place better.

Vanisha: I personally don't like the stiff carriers either because they dig into the rolls as well.

AJ: Everyone is different!

Vanisha: Absolutely, I have big boobs, right, I've said that already, but they are heavy. So if I already have my bra band digging into me, and then I put another strap on top of that, with the weight of them bearing down on it, it's going to hurt. It needs to be padded to stop the weight being so concentrated.

AJ: Another consideration, yeah.

Vanisha: My advice is always: try before you buy. And don't buy it if you don't like it! If someone wants to buy you a sling or a carrier, ask them for a voucher for your local sling library or consultant to try different slings once your baby is here, or in pregnancy with a weighted doll. It's also vastly different living with a sling day to day than it is trying it on quickly at a sling library. Sometimes people say, when they have it on in front of me, 'This is great, I love it!' Then they come back the following week or session and say, 'After 10 minutes it was hurting, I want to try something else.' Don't buy it before trying it out in your day-to-day life.

AJ: Brilliant advice!

Vanisha: I've done so many sling jobs where people come with the preconception of what they want. They want comfortable and simple so they ask around and everyone has this type of sling, so they want that one. I did a consultation once with a new mum and she was insistent that she wanted this type of sling. Put the baby in it and he said nope, almost immediately. Tried all these other slings and baby wasn't having any of it. I said, 'I did bring the bonus sling, or the mystery sling sometimes I call it, shall we try that one?' It was a ring sling.

AJ: I love ring slings, think I already said that, ha ha!

Vanisha: I love them too. But the second that baby's bum hit the little hammock on that ring sling he snuggled in. He did this little wiggle, like 'I'm a get comfy right here' and went to sleep. Sometimes what works for others isn't what works for you. I watched the mum's shoulders drop as she relaxed into it and watched her baby sigh softly and sleep. She was picking up the dog's lead and was ready to head out the door! That's what she wanted, something to pop on to take the dog out with.

AJ: I think a lot of people are put off by a ring sling because it looks complicated.

Vanisha: Oh yes!

AJ: It's very simple once you get the hang of it. It's like anything to start with, it's going to feel all fingers and thumbs, but once it clicks, it's just bliss.

Vanisha: It's a learned skill, totally.

AJ: So if you are reading this and thinking you like the look of ring slings but are put off by some folks who say it's a steep learning curve, I promise it's worth it. You will use that sling for years. I've had a baby not even an hour old in a sling and I've had my then preschooler in a sling.

Vanisha: I still use it with M, nearly six now.

AJ: It's so handy for when they reach that beautiful but frustrating stage of 'No buggy, me walk.' You get 10 paces and the 'Up!' demand comes out and you can just chuck them in and off you go. I love it. Obviously, I am hugely biased, but that's just me!

Vanisha: Also worth noting is that the same ring sling can be worn by people of very different sizes. If you have two parents, one is skinny and one is fat, it will work for both. If you find a sling that just goes wide enough for you and you grow, or your baby grows, then suddenly it's too small. A ring sling really does grow with you and your baby.

AJ: What you were saying before about watching that mum's shoulders drop as she relaxed with a sleeping baby on her chest all snuggled in the sling really panged me. I miss that, I miss that feeling that after 18 carriers and loads of sweat and sometimes tears it clicks. And you watch them physically exhale all that tension. It puts me in mind of my friend, who ran the sling library with me – I couldn't have done it without her (if you are reading this, Becci, you are a legend and I love you). Becci rang me up and said I have a friend who wants a sling but is a bit worried about coming to the session. I can't remember exactly what she said but it was along the lines of 'She's like us', meaning fat. Becci said that when she told her friend that not only was I her mate and she therefore knew I would be safe for her, but that I was also fat, she then felt able to come along and would be coming next session. And let me tell you, we got Becci's friend and her beautiful baby comfy and safe in a sling. She even walked home with the baby in the carrier while pushing the pram. She loved the feeling of her baby being so close. That's what it is about, right there. She so nearly didn't have that because she, understandably, assumed that slings and carriers are only for straight-sized people.

Oh no, I might have to start a sling library again!

Vanisha: But just goes to show the benefits of slings, how that will improve bonding and feeding!

AJ: Yes, back to feeding! A lot of what we have already covered in slings is going to be translatable to infant feeding too, right? Lack of visibility and training from the side of the birth workers or HCPs about fat folks is going to impact fat service users' self-efficacy, right?

So what needs to change in terms of lactation education and fat parents?

Vanisha: First off, let's stop assuming that everyone is a size 10 with a C cup! Let's stop assuming everyone has nipples the size of a 20p coin, stop assuming that everyone's areola is the same size. How are the mantras of infant feeding like 'Make sure most of the areola is in baby's mouth' going to translate if you have an areola the size of a dinner plate?! It's not going to work. You can have tiny breasts and huge areola; you can have massive ta tas like mine and small areola relative to nipple or breast size. This ideal of body shapes, size and proportions only works for a limited scope of parents. When I talk about shaping breasts to enable deeper latching (like the 'flipple' technique, sometimes referred to as the 'breast burger') a lot of folks will start asserting that you mustn't use your hands on your chest while feeding because it impacts latch and the like. However, if you have M cup-sized boobs and nipples that point to 7pm on the clock face rather than C cups that have a perfectly centralized 50p sized nipple, you need to shape them. You can try leaning back and putting muslins or t-shirts under the breast or chest, but that will only go so far. Putting mums and parents off using their hands to support latching might sound like a good idea in principle, but that gives no consideration to the mums and parents who have to. Cross-cradle position (baby lying on its side with its head level with the breast you are feeding from, with the parent's opposite arm holding them with baby's tummy on their parent's tummy) just won't work for some people. If you have a belly that sticks out further than your breast or chest you are not going to be able to get baby comfortably tucked into your body for baby to feed without them craning their neck.

AJ: I love koala hold (baby straddling your thigh, baby looking up at the breast) and side-lying feeding (feeding while lying down) too. Although from my lived experience and my professional experience it usually takes a week or so to nail side-lying feeding. It's a skill, isn't it?

A skill that you and your baby are learning together and that might take some time.

Vanisha: It also promotes rest and sleep in the feeding parent too!

AJ: Absolutely.

Vanisha: You also have both your hands free if you are side lying. So, for people with big boobs who need a hand free to help shape their breast or chest to get that deep latch, side lying will also support this. It also removes the weight of baby on people's stomachs. Regardless of size there are plenty of folks for whom having a baby on their stomachs in their immediate perinatal period is uncomfortable or downright painful. Side lying, again, means that the bed takes the weight of the baby and not the parent's arms or stomach.

AJ: This is all great information for the parents themselves to hear and to read. What is it that the professionals or the birth workers providing these lactation services need to know about providing support for fat parents?

Vanisha: First, check yourself. Check your bias, check your assumptions, check your blind spots. You might not even know that you are harbouring negative stereotypes or assumptions about fat people. You might be aware of your conscious bias, but it's that unconscious bias that will come up and bite your butt. No one knows everything – it's that simple. Get yourself that training. Once you are aware of the gaps in your training, then fill them. There are so many workshops and talks focusing on 'Diversity and Inclusion'; I do a cultural bias workshop.

AJ: I have done that workshop and it is fantastic!

Vanisha: Thank you.

AJ: It really did ask me so many questions that initially made me uncomfortable, for example the question about 'How white is your inner circle?' But your workshop really empowered me to ask myself those questions with the focus on the results for Black and Brown folks rather than my feelings about the answers.

Vanisha: It's the same for queer competency, right? We want folks to come and do these trainings so that LGBTQ+ people feel seen and supported.

AJ: Absolutely, and it cements again this assumption that our objection is simply and only erasure – 'Boo hoo, we feel left out' – rather than that we are systematically harmed by being left out because HCPs and birth workers don't know how to support us because we are left out. Like, how Black and Brown folks are left out of the imagery in diagnosing mastitis or blebs because the imagery and discussion is based on white folks by default.

Vanisha: This is exactly what I have tried, time and time again, to raise with communities and organizations. I got fed up in the end because I would say my piece, but no action would be taken. No changes would be made. My experience is that these resources might be out there, but you have to look hard to find them. There are trainings on Black and Brown folks breastfeeding and how the white-centric bias does a disservice to Black and Brown people. Imagine the amount of fat Black people who are looking for support and can't find it. I can't speak for the LGBTQ+ community, but again, consider fat, Black and LGBTQ+ folks, where do they go? As a professional, if you are acknowledging that you aren't the best person to offer this family that support, then you should be backing that up with 'but I know who might be able to help us'.

AJ: What resources can you recommend for parents' reading?

Vanisha: Breaking Breastfeeding Barriers & Uplifting Education gives free antenatal breastfeeding education for parents as well as training for those who would like to support breastfeeding.[8] There are also collectives like Abuela Doulas[9] that focus on Black and Brown maternal and perinatal support and education. The National Breastfeeding Helpline (0300 100 0212) is also free support that folks can access. Also, it's worth contacting your nearest professional in whatever capacity you need, like breastfeeding, chest-feeding or doula support etc., and asking them who they know about in the area.

AJ: I actively encourage people to do that on my website, like, 'If I am not the right person for you, please still get in touch if you are struggling to find what you need. I'll see who I know in your area, and I'll be glad to facilitate that sharing of resources, for sure!'

Vanisha: Absolutely.

AJ: Inevitably the conversation about referring on to other folks who might be more suited to give that care and support brings discomfort, that as birth workers we are so focused on this 'I am here to support everyone' we feel uncomfortable referring on to someone with more specialized experience or someone from within a marginalized or oppressed group of people. What would you say to those folks?

Vanisha: It's not about you. You are not for everybody, and everybody is not for you. Everyone has their own specific requirements from their birth workers. You can't be everything to all people. Your want to support people doesn't trump their right to be cared for by their kinfolk – if that is what they want.

It's not about you.

*

8   www.121doula.co.uk/services/breaking-breastfeeding-barriers-uplifting-education
9   https://abueladoulas.co.uk

I implore you, ask your training providers, your trust leaders, the people who create the resources for your service, why their imagery is restricted. Why is all the imagery straight-sized folks? Why is all the imagery of white people? Why are there no LGBTQ+ families in the imagery? Allyship doesn't have to look like caps-locked arguments on social media. Asking why our voices are missing from forums or focus groups, why our imagery and language are excluded from resources, will, arguably, have more of an impact on improving outcomes for marginalized folks than that does.

CHAPTER 14

Fat Parenting

Raising kids in a world that demonizes fat folks at worst and 'others' them at best is hard, especially as nearly all fat parents were themselves raised in a world that 'othered', shamed and devalued them because of their fat bodies. One of the things I love most (and that terrifies me the most) about parenting is the cathartic possibility to re-parent yourself. Break bits of your parenting off and feed it to your inner child. It was this very subject that started a conversation with Molly Forbes (she/her), author of *Body Happy Kids*,[1] founder of the non-profit The Body Happy Org and campaigner, which began our conversation about parenting and body image.

Interview with Molly Forbes

AJ: I do love this idea of parenting yourself a bit while parenting your kids. My parents weren't strict by any stretch of the imagination. I was a little girl in the 90s who was 'allowed' to have a short bob (still, a bob and not a short back and sides that I wanted, but it was shorter, and that alone felt like a victory). My parents did also buy me clothes from whatever section of the store I wanted, and although there was 'push-back', it was never straight-up denied. So when my kid came to me, at a similar age I was when I asked, and asked for a short back and sides, I allowed myself to break a little piece of this moment off and feed it to my inner child. I was able to say, 'Totally, it's your hair and your choice, buddy. And if you don't like it: hair grows!'

---

1   www.bodyhappyorg.com/shop/body-happy-kids-book

Molly: Absolutely, and a lot of parents are coming to this work because they want to try and ensure that their kids don't feel the way they felt or feel still about their bodies. Or they are becoming aware of how prevalent body shaming is among young people and they are really shocked. It is totally understandable that they will come at it from a [child-centred] angle, but it's important for parents to know that they may have an amount of unlearning to do themselves first. Not to say that they must be an expert and have everything figured out, especially as our relationship with our bodies changes over time – it is not a linear thing. But you can't jump to raising kids who are at home and confident in their bodies if you are still holding those biases about your body or the bodies of people around you.

There are different layers to this conversation. First, if you have been subjected to weight stigma and you have been subjected to anti-fat bias, or you have been shamed and told that your body is 'wrong' your entire life, you are going to carry so many feelings and thought processes about living in a fat body. It is understandable that parents want to protect their kids from experiencing this. This can play out in them trying to change their kids' bodies. They don't want their kids to experience the same type of anti-fat discrimination and prejudice that they have experienced, so their way of ensuring that doesn't happen is to attempt to change their kids.

AJ: Rather than the system or the societal and individual view of fatness, right?

Molly: Yes. We know that weight is complex, and weight is not an indicator of health. This idea that you can change your body like you change your outfit is just not true.

AJ: I had this conversation with Nicola Salmon!

Molly: Yes!

AJ: That in, not totally all, because there will be pedants, but in nearly all cases, you can't change your body, so Nicola asks, 'What would happen if you stayed exactly as you are?'!

Molly: We are taught that our weight is a direct indication of our health, and that our weight is all within our individual control, if we just eat the 'right' food or move our body in the 'right' way. We're taught not to trust our bodies, to constantly survey and monitor them, and to restrict all the time. And this then impacts how we approach our kids' bodies too. Society teaches us to inherently not trust kids' bodies. We don't trust when kids are hungry, what they need to eat etc. We don't trust when they will be ready to potty train or use the toilet etc. We just inherently don't trust them to know their bodies. We also don't trust adults to know their bodies, especially people who are giving birth. This model of not trusting people to know their bodies has permeated through a lot of the healthcare system.

AJ: Ask a doula, any doula, or gestational parent if they have a story about people knowing their bodies and labours and it being dismissed; we all have one, or seventeen thousand examples of this. It's true!

Molly: There is a real distrust from the 'system' that kids know how much to move their bodies, or how to move their bodies, and what to eat and what to seek out in terms of variety of foods etc. that we end up with kids on eating plans and exercise plans to try and change their bodies. And because there are so many factors that influence the shape of our bodies and how we look, these plans inevitably fail. They cause harm, either through body esteem disruption or a messed-up relationship with food. And they cause a huge amount of shame, too. And all of this perpetuates the distrust in kids' bodies – and makes them not trust their own bodies either. This is not just happening through the way food or bodies might be talked about at home, but also in the way this stuff is approached by the medical professionals around them, the teachers and other family such as grandparents. It's unsurprising, then, that kids as young as three can show anti-fat bias or say that there is something 'wrong' with fat bodies. It is not just this thing that happens to teenagers. Traditionally we have always thought of poor body image as something that happens to teenage girls, and we know that's not true. Poor body image can impact kids of all ages and genders.

There is another layer, too. When a child is considered to fall outside of our society's narrow view of what is an 'acceptable body', then the parents often get judged. Often there's an assumption that the parents are lazy or uneducated or are simply feeding their kids the 'wrong' foods. We hear these classist tropes happening all the time in the way the media talks about parents and in the way public health policies often focus on educating parents about nutrition – assuming that a parent who has a fat child does not know the nutritional value of vegetables.

Parents are under a huge amount of pressure to make their children's bodies conform to what our society deems as an acceptable body. Also, the parent might be living in a fat body themselves, and may have been dealing with weight stigma and anti-fat bias their whole lives, too. They have been told their own body is wrong, or that not only are they 'not looking after' their own health; they're also not looking after their child's health. All of this creates fear, shame and a culture that makes it very hard for children simply to be at peace in their bodies. Rather than giving kids the message that some bodies are good and some are bad, we should be helping them to know, intrinsically, that bodies exist on a spectrum: there is no such thing as a good or bad body, there is no wrong way to have a body.

Unfortunately, this distrust and body shame and fear of fatness starts really young. For example, a parent takes their baby to be weighed at a baby clinic, and they are told, 'Your baby is on the 95th – or higher – centile, you need to monitor their feeds and make sure you're not over-feeding them.' Then, when the child is a bit older, they take them to the nurse for something else and they are told again, 'Your child is too heavy; you need to cut out snacks or increase the amount of movement that your child is doing.' We are again fostering this belief that teachers, healthcare professionals, elders etc., anyone with perceived 'authority' over our bodies, know our bodies better than we know them. And then later, when the child starts primary school, they are weighed in Reception and again in Year 6, and might get a letter home saying their weight is too high. They aren't just getting these messages about bodies on social media – they're getting them from people in positions of authority, from the most trusted adults in their lives. We are setting children and young people up to have the most difficult time possible in trying to love and accept their bodies – *and* all the bodies of those around them.

It's hard to see how people come through this system with anything other than a deep misunderstanding and anti-fat-biased view of their own and other bodies. Parents then need to unlearn all this messaging that they have absorbed their entire lives that their body is wrong. It's a gargantuan task. There is a huge temptation to blame social media for the poor body image that many young people experience, and don't get me wrong, social media does play a role. But we need to look at the messaging that they are getting before they even have social media accounts. This is the base coding for poor body image. By the time kids are using social media they already have really entrenched views of what counts as a good body and what a bad body looks like. These views have come from the people closest to them and people in positions of authority around them.

AJ: It also, I think, prioritizes being in an 'acceptable' body over health, because you can't tell if someone is healthy or not by looking at them, and health and weight are not paired factors. So often the priority is to 'look' healthy: straight sized. This is one of the reasons, when I saw your most recent post, the one about weighing kids in school and what that does to children and what it doesn't do to their health, I knew we needed to have this conversation. I have opted my kids out of being weighed at school since they started school. In fact, I used to take them out of school on the day I knew it was happening because as a parent of a disabled child, I had to consider the possibility of them not being listened to or being coerced into being weighed against their will. Especially when you consider you are then told, among your peers in some circumstances, if you are healthy or unhealthy based on an equation from hundreds of years ago based on eugenics, white supremacy and misogyny...how do we even attempt to undo that base coding of BMI = health when this is the deal for primary-age kids! It's mind-boggling.

Molly: The National Child Measurement Programme means that a nurse will come in when your child is in Reception and Year 6 and weigh them, unless you specifically opt out. (You used to have to give consent, but the GDPR (General Data Protection Regulation) changes in 2018 meant the consent was flipped, so now you have to opt out instead of opting in.)

Lots of nurses don't like the weighing aspect of the programme or the focus on weight, and often it's not nurses who actually implement the programme but healthcare assistants instead. A really good way to look at it is that it has nothing to do with health, and everything to do with politics. It is interesting to think about where the programme came from, as this can help us understand that many of these health policies aren't really about health at all. We need to ask, who is advising the government about these policies? What organization and companies are benefiting from the vilification of fatness and the weight normative approach to health that we have in this country?

AJ: I am going to butcher your words here as I can't recall verbatim, but you said something along the lines of 'the National Child Measurement Programme isn't proven to improve outcomes' – if we take 'improve' to mean reduce the BMI of our society.

Molly: It doesn't make us thin! Weighing children in schools does not make them thin. And actually, the focus on kids' weight is not helpful at all – not if we really, genuinely, care about health. As long as we can say that health is an individual thing, it lets the government off the hook. If you just eat the right foods, cook from scratch, move your body enough, if we put all the onus onto the people, then the government cannot be accountable for falling health inequalities. They don't have to invest in reducing inequality or weight stigma or improve access to public healthcare for all. It's much easier to just tell everyone to go on a diet.

AJ: Does it tie in with the view that we have a whole generation or a whole segment of society that has been so busy and focused on making themselves smaller? Smaller in their bodies, smaller in their sexuality or gender identity, smaller and smaller, just shush, right? This is primarily, of course, women and people assigned female at birth. Then they have less time to fuck shit up? Less time to disrupt the systems of oppression and disparities of health outcomes, social outcomes, social economic outcomes, and all the rest of it?

Molly: It's so ableist, too. On the face of it, they might justify it as 'Oh, we just want kids to be healthy and eat the right foods, and we're just looking out for kids' health.' What does that say to disabled kids and disabled people? If health is this unobtainable goal that disabled people can never reach because they are living with conditions that mean that our society's definition of health will forever be inaccessible to them...what does that say about their worth as human beings in society? That they are less valuable? Less important? This is why it is so important to examine the roots of these systems. They are rooted in ableism, white supremacy and hierarchical views of bodies. *You cannot separate the pursuit of the perfect body from the vilification of 'othered' bodies.* They are two sides of the same coin. You can't say that you shouldn't just want to be thin like supermodels while also saying, 'Don't be fat, it's unhealthy' – those two messages don't mix. When I grew up in the 90s, diet culture was presented in a very different way; it was very obviously diet culture. But now, the world that my children are growing up in, it can be much harder to spot. We have become wise to the fact that diets don't work and that diet culture is negative. So it's morphed into 'wellness' or 'healthism', and by extension the idea that health = worth. It's just another way to put bodies into a hierarchy. (Of course, however it's packaged, all the bodies we are told are healthy only look one way, and the wellness eating plans are all diets. Just look at how WeightWatchers is now Wellness Watchers. That says everything you need to know really.)

AJ: Arg, I can't remember where I saw it but I saw someone clarify it as WeightWatchers having a midlife crisis. They have realized that a lot of people are rightly wary of diets and diet culture because it often actually causes people to be heavier than when they started, and the stress of weight cycling on the body etc., more and more people are aware of the effects of diet culture than ever before, so they have tried the leather jacket and the convertible plan and rebranded as 'Wellness Watchers'!

Molly: Exactly. They need people through the doors and so they have tried to make diet culture harder to spot by rebranding it as 'wellness' or 'lifestyle changes'. The easy way to spot it is, if the aim is weight loss, then it's a diet. It's diet culture. It doesn't matter how you phrase it or how you package it – if the ultimate aim of the game is intentional weight loss...then it's diet culture. Perhaps a better name for it is anti-fat culture, because this clearly labels it for what it is. As always, it's interesting to look at the financial incentives of viewing health this way. Who are the companies benefiting from this approach to health? Who are the companies getting a lot of money from NHS contracts to provide weight management services, for example? Which companies might benefit from schemes that see GP surgeries incentivized for referrals of patients to them? This is all-important to keep in mind when we're looking at the bigger picture here.

AJ: Because the aim is to lose weight first and foremost, not necessarily to be healthier.

Molly: Yes, because the thought process is, if people are thinner, then there will be less strain on the NHS. But if you look at how much money is being directed into these services, it's not making people thinner or healthier. They just lead to people weight cycling – all the evidence shows that, long term, most people don't lose weight and keep the weight off. And this weight cycling (plus the impact of weight stigma) is independently bad for health.

So who is benefiting from this arrangement? The NHS? The service users? The 'weight management services'? And what is the cost of all the children and young people currently on pathways or waiting lists for treatment for eating disorders and disordered eating? The amount of children and young people seeking treatment for eating disorders or disordered eating is at the highest it's ever been. The NHS cannot treat this amount of people; it is simply not able to do so. What is the cost of all these young people experiencing eating disorders or disordered eating on the NHS? What is the cost of that emotionally and physically for them and their families and wider circles? Could funding of weight management services be better directed to other services?

AJ: Again, it comes back to the position of worthiness. If you are in a fatter body, you are costing the NHS money, so you are less worthy of treatment. Like what I am living through right now, not being able to find a surgeon who will remove my gallbladder. So then my treatment takes longer, and I require further investigations; more emergency care is then sought because the pain becomes unmanageable, or the condition can even worsen and require emergency surgery or complications that require further surgery or additional treatment compared to whipping the problematic organ out as promptly as would have happened for a straight-sized person. That's surely a factor of why my care is costing more than just purely 'I am fat, and I am taking up too much space and funding.'

Molly: We know that anti-fat bias shows up in doctors and other healthcare professionals, and we know that means that fat people put off going to the doctor. We can view that as a symptom of a fatphobic system that by the time fat people come to the system, they are likely to be further along in their condition, or the condition has worsened because they have put off treatment. That is another reason why it might, comparatively, be more expensive than a straight-sized person's care. It also doesn't look at the health inequality causes. Over 4 million children in the UK are currently experiencing food poverty.[2]

AJ: What do you say to parents, then, who are starting their fat neutrality or body neutrality journey? Apart from reading *Body Happy Kids* of course!

Molly: The first thing is to recognize that none of this (anti-fat bias, diet culture, fatphobia, the lot) is one individual's fault. It is a systemic issue, and we need to challenge the culture. Having said that, we are all individuals within this culture, so we do have a role to play. Second, it doesn't happen overnight. These ideas are so deeply ingrained, and if you have grown up being told, your entire life, that your body is wrong or certain foods are wrong, you can't suddenly wake up one day and change that. The responsibility shouldn't have to be on you as an individual to have to unlearn all of these fatphobic tropes or biases; the responsibility should be on society to not teach that only certain bodies are good bodies and only some foods are good foods. It can be very scary to come face to face with this discussion, though. There are people who have spent their entire lives invested in the pursuit of thinness, so it's a big thing to give that up, especially if giving it up means they may be treated even more badly by the people and systems around them. This is compounded by the fact we often equate thinness with success and fatness with failure in our culture. It is difficult to give up those ideals. So be kind to yourself, take extra care of yourself during this process, and acknowledge that this is difficult and messy and not straightforward.

It can help to start small, simply by changing the way you talk about bodies, movement, health and food with your children – or even just stop talking about this stuff at all. If you can't be neutral, just try not to say anything at all.

I also think it's important to neutralize the language we use around food, bodies, movement – all of it. And use the word 'fat' as the neutral

---

2   https://commonslibrary.parliament.uk/research-briefings/cbp-9209

descriptor that it is (we don't use other words for tall or short or thin, and finding other words for fat can end up just perpetuating the idea it's a bad word and a bad type of body to have).

Help your kids develop their media literacy skills and have conversations about this stuff from a young age. This stuff shows up in kids' media right from day one – just think of *Peppa Pig* and how Daddy Pig's fat tummy is often the punchline of the joke.

Dropping the morality from food can also be a good starting point. For example: 'Oh you've been very good and eaten all your vegetables even though they are yucky, so now we can be naughty and have some chocolate – but only a little bit because it's bad for us and we don't want to get fat!' Don't do that!

Also start to think about your boundaries for other people around you and your children as well. For example:

> We know that Aunty Bethel has a really different way of talking and thinking about food and bodies, so she might say something about some foods being bad and some being good. Or she might talk about your body or my body and comment her thoughts about us, what we eat, how much we move and our health. She's doing it the old way, we're doing it a new way, and we are allowed to say 'no' to her comments on our bodies or how we think, talk and feel about food.

AJ: That would be a great conversation to have before school as well I think, because even my straight-sized kid has been called fat as an insult, before they were in Juniors, I think; they were still in Infants.

Molly: The temptation is to say, 'Oh, you're not fat you are beautiful', but this gives the power back to fat as an unbeautiful or undesirable thing. We can say, 'I can see why that hurt your feelings' and we can listen and validate without giving in to the temptation to move away from fat as a neutral descriptor. Of course, we want our children to be healthy and happy and all those things, but we also don't want them to have to go back and unlearn, like many of us have had to, all these toxic and unhealthy manifestations of diet culture and anti-fat bias.

It isn't just about them, though; if we model to them that they are worthy of respect, dignity and love regardless of their body size, then they are going to be good humans who see others who are also worthy of respect, dignity and love, regardless of how their bodies look and regardless of how their bodies function.

This point of 'everyone is worthy' is where a lot of people realize that this is a social justice issue. It is a social justice issue because we have people who are being denied healthcare, dying waiting for healthcare, or dying being refused healthcare based on their BMI. Which is unacceptable. If we want to raise anti-racist children, we need to talk to them about racism. If we want to raise non-ableist children, talk to them about ableism. So we need to talk to them about fatphobia, weight bias or weight stigma, too. How those conversations happen will depend on many factors, namely their age and where you, as the parent, are at in your own journey, but starting small with removing morality from food will have a huge impact on the way you and your children view food, so their building blocks of morality and worth won't include food or weight. That is a huge gift to give to the next generation.

AJ: Another way that I was able to rewrite the parenting around bodies and feed a little bit of it back to my inner child is when my kids ask to jiggle my belly! When we are rough housing or whatever on the floor and they ask for raspberries or tickles, and they want to do it back to me and they say, 'Your belly is so jiggly and soft!', rather than snatching my t-shirt back down and being hurt I say, 'Yeah!!! It's so soft, it's so jiggly isn't it!' and they try to do raspberries, but they can't because they are laughing too hard and then we all have a cuddle! That feels incredibly empowering to allow myself to hear their words as positive.

Molly: That is a moment of pure joy. Living in this world, among all these horrors. We don't have to live a joyless existence. We are allowed happiness and joy.

CHAPTER 15

Rebuttals, Objections and Advocacy

Thinking long and hard about how to end this book, I arrived at the conclusion that the most valuable parting information might be some of the 'sound bites' I have picked up from my birth and postnatal doula training, personal and professional experience, as well as from spending time in the presence of so many incredible and experienced birth workers who bring generations of not only wisdom, but also insider information on how to best navigate the system.

I remember hearing about midwife Mary Cronk's phrasebook for the first time while training with Abuela Doulas (the UK's first Black-founded and Black-run doula training school, and one of the few that is an actively safe space for trans and non-binary doulas). Coach, Doula Trainer and birth advocate, Mars Lord was speaking to us about times where our clients may want us to use our voice to help them be heard. Although a lot of people think, understandably, given the poor examples of doulas that are often in the media (people over-stepping and putting their views ahead of their clients' wishes), that a doula's job is to speak for their client, most of the work that doulas and other birth workers do is in the prep. (I have been contacted on the Wednesday, interviewed on the Friday, paid on the Saturday and been at the birth Sunday evening before, so it's not always the case.) The 'prep' may look like asking questions such as 'Is there a point at which you want me to speak up?' For example, when I am caring for trans and non-binary clients, I ask them if or when they would like me to intervene if someone is misgendering them or using language that they have already asked HCPs not to use. Everybody is different; some people will say, 'I want you to speak up every time' and others will say, 'Wait for me to give you the signal' – this can be verbal or non-verbal; usually it's a look that just screams, 'You are being subbed in mate, wade in!' So if you are supporting your loved one, or you are speaking with your loved one about how they can best support you, consider how you would feel best supported. Do you want them to stand behind you and be witness to you and your words? Or do you want them to stand in front of you and speak for you? It may be a mixture of these approaches based on what is happening at the time. It is worth considering and discussing this in advance, particularly for people who are outside of the expected maternity or perinatal service users, such as fat people, LGBTQ+ people, Black and Brown people or disabled people.

Some of my favourite work is relaying some of these 'sound bites' or 'phrase book' entries that can help remind everyone in earshot that this is the service user's show. This is their body, their baby and their fucking choice.

I have used many of these in multiple settings – from when my late grandmother broke her hip and her position in the surgery queue kept being leap frogged:

> I thought that the outcomes for hip break patients dropped dramatically at 72 hours (I already looked this up). I am sure there must be a very good reason she keeps getting moved, and I appreciate it's not your fault. However, I am worried about the potential of a negative outcome based on these delays. Would you mind giving me your name and pin number[1] in case I need to come back to the issue later?

Surgery happened a few hours later.

I used many of them on many occasions when my late father was

---

1   A 'pin' number is a unique number that is issued to members of medical professional bodies including the Nursing and Midwifery Council (NMC) and General Medical Council (GMC).

admitted to hospital. And, of course, I have used them as a parent to advocate for my children when I felt their autonomy was being diminished or their voice was being ignored.

Mary Cronk's phrasebook reads:

1. 'Thank you so much Midwife Sinister/ Mr Hi-an-my-tee, for your *advice*. We will consider this carefully and let you know our *decision*.' Sweet smile! *This one is most useful in the antenatal stage, although it can be used in labour. It can just take a minute to consider what you either want to know, or what you decide.*

2. 'Would you like to reconsider what you have just said!' Fierce glare. *This is useful and, for example, applies to the misuse of the word 'allow'.*

3. 'I do not believe you can have heard what I have just said. Shall I repeat myself?'

4. 'I am afraid I will have to regard any further discussion as harassment.' *This is used if the person does not respect your decision or persists in pressing the subject.*

5. 'What is your NMC or GMC pin number?' *This is used if no. 4 is ineffective. If the person asks why you want their pin number, inform them that this is something they might like to consider.*

6. 'STOP THIS AT ONCE!' *This is to be used in extremis. I am delighted to tell you that this was used AGAINST me by a woman to whom I had taught it. I was doing a difficult VE (vaginal examination) and was being too persistent. I stopped at once and learned a lesson.*

Some of my staples are variations on these headers. Finding how you best, organically, speak these phrases is important. There is no point memorizing them if they don't feel organic for you as the service user or indeed as a support person who, with permission from the service user, may need to employ some of these objections yourself. Some people prefer the direct and succinct approach, and others find that 'playing dumb' works best for them. I personally think that the more options or skill sets you have in your quiver, the better. The purpose of these phrases is often to disrupt what is currently happening or being proposed and to remind everyone in the room of the autonomy and rights of the service user. It is unfortunately a case of knowing the right buzz word sometimes – like when filling out a form that you know isn't going to be read by a human but will be scanned by a computer looking for key phrases and terminology, sometimes we have to take this approach with communication in these instances.

Saying 'I feel rushed' or 'pushed' might not have the same effect as saying 'I feel coerced'. All words, by all people, should be heard, respected and acted on, but sadly, this often isn't the case.

One of my most commonly used disrupting sound bites is to ask the service user, 'Do you have any more questions you'd like to ask before you make your decision?' or, 'Have you been given all the information you need so that you can make your decision?' This serves to remind and refocus everyone in the room or in the discussion of the service user's absolute autonomy in treatment. Failing this, or in addition, if I can sense that my service user is feeling rushed or on the spot, I have employed 'Do you want time to consider your options? Remember, you don't have to answer now, you are allowed to take time to make your decision...' Usually, the first disruption is enough, but I have had to employ the second for a client I was supporting who was planning a breech vaginal delivery. The first objection didn't seem to land with the obstetrician, but once I had laboured the 'You are allowed to take time to consider *your* options about *your* labour and *your* baby', she did offer a quiet room for discussion and reflection on the service user's options with her support people (her husband and me) before proceeding.

A disrupter method that I have used in all sorts of circumstances is one I learned from Mars Lord: confirm back to the person what they have said. For example, if you are, as a fat parent, told that you 'must' give birth at the hospital, then mirroring back what they have asserted as fact can sometimes nudge them to reconsider how they have phrased their assertion. For example: 'Could I just confirm what you have said here...you said I *must* have my baby in hospital? Are you saying that I don't have a choice about where I birth my baby?'

If, after being given an opportunity to reflect on their phrasing they are still asserting that you do not have autonomy or choice, you could ask them to record their assertion in your notes. For example: 'Could you write down in my notes that you have told me I cannot decline to be induced today, please', and in particular situations you may want to ask them, as Mary Cronk's point 5 does, to also ensure they put their pin number alongside their notes.

Similarly for situations of your BMI being used to gatekeep services, feel free to ask for written confirmation of your BMI being the deciding factor. For example, if you are told that you cannot be referred to conception assistance based on your BMI, asking the HCP to document that on the system or notes might spur reflection and/or reconsideration from the HCP: 'Can you record in my notes that the reason I can't be referred is my BMI please.' Or, if this feels uncomfortable, perhaps use 'Could I just confirm, so I've got it right, that what are you saying is that because of my BMI I cannot access this service?'

Mary Cronk's phrasebook entry 6 'STOP THIS AT ONCE!' is mighty effective. As a support person you may want to employ similar phrases that once again remind all in earshot that the autonomy and consent of the service user is king. For example: 'THEY HAVE SAID STOP', or additionally phrases such as 'I do not consent, treating me without consent (or after I have withdrawn it) is assault. Stop. Now.'

'I do not consent' is a phrase that, sadly, I think, needs to be shown to all people entering any medical setting. I have taught this phrase to my children and will go over it with my doula clients because 'no' or 'stop' sadly sometimes don't seem to cut through once the motions are in full flow.

Sometimes not being heard might take the shape of asking you to reconsider an intervention that you have already declined. It might sound like 'I know at previous appointments you have declined being weighed, but I thought I would ask you again because it is really important, and you might reconsider.' A simple 'I have answered that question already' might be sufficient, but in situations of overt insistences, 'Could you ensure that my response to this question has been documented? People keep asking me questions I've already answered, and not only is it a waste of your time and mine, but this feels like bullying now.' Or more directly: 'I have declined this already; repeated questioning of my decisions is coercion. Please stop.'

The idea isn't to hold the threat of litigation over the heads of HCPs, but to disrupt the trajectory of the coercion, lack of bodily autonomy or human rights infringements that might, and soberingly does, happen.

The overwhelming majority, or maybe more accurately nearly all HCPs, I say fairly confidently, don't spend years of study while getting into tens of thousands in debt just to be horrible to people. I don't doubt for a second the conviction and dedication to uphold the human rights and bodily autonomy of all who birth that most HCPs display. It is necessary, however, to sometimes remind people of these immutable rights. Pregnancy, labour and the perinatal period is a relatively short period, which, for most people, means the most interactions in a short space of time that they have had with HCPs. It might also be the first time that service users have been admitted to hospital or seen a consultant. As birth was taken from community teams and further back, from granny midwives, it has been more and more medicalized. The central pillars of autonomy and choice are often diminished or held in equal stead to policy and protocol. Remember that their policy ain't your policy. Hospital policy might say 'No eating on the labour ward'; your policy might be, and is allowed to be, 'I eat when I am hungry.' And honestly? I am the same!

We can look at any trust in the UK, or indeed at the wider world, at the mode of birth stats, and see that birth is becoming more medicalized. A report from the World Health Organization (WHO) on caesarean sections rates states:

According to new research from the World Health Organization (WHO), caesarean section use continues to rise globally, now accounting for more than 1 in 5 (21%) of all childbirths. This number is set to continue increasing over the coming decade, with nearly a third (29%) of all births likely to take place by caesarean section by 2030, the research finds. While a caesarean section can be an essential and lifesaving surgery, it can put women and babies at unnecessary risk of short- and long-term health problems if performed when there is not medical need.

'Caesarean sections are absolutely critical to save lives in situations where vaginal deliveries would pose risks, so all health systems must ensure timely access for all women when needed,' said Dr Ian Askew, Director of WHO's Department of Sexual and Reproductive Health and Research and the UN joint programme, HRP. 'But not all the caesarean sections carried out at the moment are needed for medical reasons. Unnecessary surgical procedures can be harmful, both for a woman and her baby.'[2]

NHS maternity statistics for 2021–22 also confirm:

Spontaneous method of onset is most common as a proportion of total deliveries but has decreased from *66 per cent* in 2011–12 to *47 per cent* in 2021–22. Caesarean method of onset increased from *12 per cent* to *20 per cent* and induced method of onset from *22 per cent* to *33 per cent* in the period 2011–12 to 2021–22.[3]

These increasing induction and caesarean birth trends have happened at the same time as an increase in maternal deaths in the UK, although, of course, correlation doesn't always equal causation. However, the MBRRACE-UK report in 2022[4] found that Black women are 3.7 times more likely to die than white women. And Asian women are 1.8 more times likely to die than white women. Also, women from deprived areas are up to 2.5 times more likely to die than those in the least deprived areas. The overall figure of women during pregnancy or up to six weeks after birth was 229. This is 24 per cent higher than 2019–20.

I don't include this information to scare you stiff about giving

---

2   www.who.int/news/item/16-06-2021-caesarean-section-rates-continue-to-rise-amid-growing-inequalities-in-access

3   https://digital.nhs.uk/data-and-information/publications/statistical/nhs-maternity-statistics/2021-22#, p.11.

4   www.npeu.ox.ac.uk/assets/downloads/mbrrace-uk/reports/maternal-report-2022/MBRRACE-UK_Maternal_Report_2022_-_Lay_Summary_v10.pdf

birth. The statistical likelihood is that you are likely to have a straight-forward pregnancy, birth and perinatal period. It is, however, worth being aware of the increasing interventions and medicalization of birth in the UK to be able to make an informed decision as to whether you wish to engage with that system. You are also free to choose to engage with just parts of that system. I have known people who have found comfort and safety in deciding their own boundaries in care that they would accept. For example, some people decline certain elements of the standard care pathway, such as growth scans or Glucose Tolerance Tests (GTTs) (as I did). It is not true that seeking midwifery care at all means that you are then confined by the system, and that you must accept any and all interventions of investigations you are offered. (Gosh, I am a broken record!)

Your pregnancy and your birth are just that. Yours. That experience belongs to you. It is likely to be an experience that will stay with you. It has the potential, as my two polar opposite births did, to change you, to move you and to empower you greatly. After birthing Emma at home into the water I felt as if I could have lifted the house from its footings and carried the whole house across town to my dad's garden so he could see his baby in their most powerful state, holding their baby.

As a doula I have had the highest privilege of watching other people have their moment. I have seen this moment play out in bedrooms, bathrooms, front rooms, birthing suits, delivery units and operating theatres. Yet still, every fucking time, I can't believe I get to love you and be here with you while you experience the biggest day of your life. Usually followed a few hours, or days, later by 'I can't believe I got to be in the room when an entire new human being joined the world.'

Wherever, and however, through your discussions and birth plan explorations you decide you want your baby to enter the world, I hope it brings you everything you need it to.

For the second + time parents it might bring you healing and validation after your first experience. Or for the first-time + parents it may solidify your belief in your incredible, remarkable, strong, capable, magic, fat body.

To close I want to remind you of the incredible wisdom that has been shared by all I have spoken to during this journey. Especially if you want to come back for a reminder during your journey!

Fiona wrote: 'I will never forget what my body did for us, what *I* did. This is the body that my daughter will remember holding her, feeding her, pushing her on the swing. This is the body that she rode around the living room like a bucking bronco and that chased her around the park. This body is her mother, and her mother is a fat old woman. And there's nothing more powerful than that.'

Nicole spoke the truth when she said: 'We are born worthy. We are inherently worthy of every bit of care, support, tests, treatment or love that people need to grow their families. I wish that people knew that and could really embody that. Your body is capable of phenomenal things.'

Caprice said, with her whole self: 'It's also important for me to pass on to other Black, fat, pregnant women and people to look at your elders, look at your families. See what the women in your family look like, what our bodies look like. It can be so far removed from the whitewashed imagery that we see surrounding pregnancy and motherhood. Seek out those safe spaces where you can be you. Oh, and eat the Puff-Puff! Enjoy your jollof rice! Don't not eat the chicken! Eat the foods we've always eaten, for your body, and for your soul!'

Dr Greenfield told us the data says: 'most women who are over-weight have a straightforward pregnancy and birth. Remember it is your job to advocate for them so they can be part of that majority.'

Amber rightly pointed out: 'If you Google "fertility symbols" or "carvings like fertility goddesses' statues" or historical "mother" pieces – they are usually fat. These totemic sculptures from ancient civilizations are, usually, voluptuous: big thighs, big bums, big bellies, big boobs! Where did that change? When did that stop? We have this modern idea of health and fertility as straight sized. If these artefacts are showing us what a fertility goddesses look like, and if this is what pregnancy and fertility looks like, then hell, I am there!'

Kate succinctly summed it all up when she said: 'Your body size doesn't change your worth.'

Orla reminded us: 'Don't wait for anyone to give you permission. Take your autonomy and don't wait for a clinician or a healthcare professional to give it to you.'

Vanisha reminded the birth workers reading this: 'It's not about you. You are not for everybody, and everybody is not for you. Everyone has their own specific requirements from their birth workers. You can't be everything to all people. Your want to support people doesn't trump their right to be cared for by their kinfolk – if that is what they want.'

And Molly finishes up with her reminder: 'We don't have to live a joyless existence. We are allowed happiness and joy.'

A final reminder from me: you aren't asking too much. You aren't being awkward or being a 'birth bitch' or any other misogynistic catchphrase that is lobbed at you. You are in charge!

It's your fucking show!

Afterword

19th June 2023

Shortly after I sent my manuscript over to JKP, I got the call I had been waiting for.

My surgery had been booked and this saga was finally coming to an end.

Apart from the first date being cancelled as I sat in the day surgery ward in my surgical stockings, and of course, the lack of appropriately sized disposable pants available, the surgery and first weeks of recovery have been uncomplicated.

Looking forward to never having a gallbladder flare-up again!

Just over three years from start to finish, with countless sleepless, painfilled nights. I did in that time manage to write this book, connect with incredible people who encouraged me to seek help or told me to go back and speak to them again, and reassured me that my mass held no bearing on my worthiness to treatment.

Very sadly, I wasn't allowed to keep my gallbladder. I wanted it ensconced in Perspex® as a trophy. A trophy that would remind me how strong my body and mind are and serve as a reminder to never doubt my worthiness of access, treatment and love again.

Perhaps I should have popped it in a box and sent it directly to the consultant who told me, 'Don't be a mother, an author, or a wife, just focus on losing 30kg. Then we can operate.'

Yeah, I should have sent it to him...

Index

AIMS Guide to Your Rights in Pregnancy and Birth, The (Ashworth) 153, 160
Am I Allowed? What Every Woman Should Know BEFORE She Gives Birth (Beech) 106
Ashworth, Emma 153

baby carriers 104, 181–5, 186, 188
Beech, Beverley Ann Lawrence 106
Belly of the Beast (Harrison) 55
Big Birthas 49, 79, 80, 83, 110, 112, 115, 120, 121–2, 128
birth
  birth plans 73, 89–90, 101, 108–9, 158–9
  and BMI 146–9, 150, 151, 152, 154
  Fiona Houston's experience of 38–41
  home births 150–9
  induced birth 81–2, 160–76
  interview with Amber Marshall 112, 118–19, 123
  medicalisation of 211–13
  rights in 106–9
  water births 80–1, 118–19, 145–9
birth plans 73, 89–90, 101, 108–9, 158–9
BJOG: An International Journal of Obstetrics & Gynaecology 155
black women
  and babywear 183–4
  experience of Fiona Houston 34–48
Body Happy Kids (Forbes) 194
body mass index (BMI)

and author's experience of maternity/perinatal services 16–21, 25–6
and conception 49–51, 53–4, 55, 56, 57–8, 59, 60, 63, 66, 70–1
and gestational diabetes 134, 135–6
and healthcare services 84–6, 210
and home births 150, 151, 152, 154
as measurement of weight 15–16, 84
and maternity/perinatal services 74–6, 84–6, 106–7
and water births 146–9
breastfeeding 72–3, 177–9, 180–1, 184–5, 188–90, 191–2
Brown, L 146

Cadwell, Karin 178
Centers for Disease Control and Prevention (CDC) 136
clothing
  interview with Amber Marshall 115–18, 128
  interview with Caprice Fox 78
  interview with Mari Greenfield 87
  interview with Nicola Salmon 64–5
  interview with Orla Gallagher 104–5
  interview with Vanisha Virgo 180–1
Cochrane Review 26, 163
conception
  and BMI 49–51, 53–4, 55, 56, 57–8, 59, 60, 63, 66, 70–1

conception *cont.*
  interview with Nico-
    la Salmon 51–65
  and IVF 49–50, 63
Cronk, Mary 206, 208, 210
cyclic obesity/ weight-based stigma
  (COBWEBS) model 27, 29, 31–3

Diabetes UK 15, 136
diabetes, gestational 134–44
dieting
  ineffectiveness of 28–9
  during pregnancy 79–80

fat
  as descriptor 12–13
  language of 11–14
  levels of fatness 13–14
Fat Birth (Mayefske) 62
Fat and Fertile (Salmon) 51
fatphobia *see also* weight stigma
  and author's experience of 16–26
  and conception 51–65
  impact of 12–13, 14–15, 16–17
  intersectionality of 14–15
  interview with Nico-
    la Salmon 51–65
  and parenting 195–205
  racism in 55
Fearing the Black Body (String) 55
Forbes, Molly
  interview with 194–205, 215
Fox, Caprice
  interview with 66–78, 214

Gallagher, Orla
  interview with 88–105, 215
Garland, D 146
gestational diabetes 134–44
Gestational Diabetes (Hughes) 135
Gestational Diabetes UK 142
Greenfield, Mari
  interview with 79–87, 214

Haddad, F 146
Hagen, Sophie 19
Harrison, Da'Shaun L. 55

healthcare services
  and BMI 84–5, 210
  weight stigma in 26–9,
    57, 61–2, 200–5
'Healthy weight' document
  (NHS Highland) 30–1
home births 150–9
Houston, Fiona
  experiences of 34–48, 214
Hughes, Deborah 135

induced birth 81–2, 160–76
Inducing Labour (Wickham) 161
intersectionality of fatphobia 14–15
IVF 49–50, 63

Kay, Adam 108

language
  of fatness 11–14
  inclusive 9–10
  interview with Caprice Fox 66–8
Lesbemums 165
levels of fatness 13–14
Lord, Mars 183, 206, 209

Mann, Traci 28–9
Marshall, Amber
  interview with 111–33, 215
  on water births 146–8
*Maternity Matters: Choice, Access and
  Continuity of Care in a Safe Service*
  (Department of Health) 150
maternity/perinatal services
  author's experience of 16–21, 25–6
  and BMI 74–6, 84–6, 106–7, 111,
    112, 114, 121, 124–6, 128–9, 130–1
  Fiona Houston's expe-
    rience of 34–48
  interview with Amber
    Marshall 111–32
  interview with Caprice Fox 68–78
  interview with Mari
    Greenfield 80–7
  interview with Orla Gal-
    lagher 89–105

and Midwifery Continuity
of Carer (MCoC) 26–7
rights in 106–9
weight stigma in 29–33, 55
working with 206–13
Mayefske, Michelle 62
MBRRACE-UK report 212
medicalisation of birth 211–13
Midwifery Continuity of
Carer (MCoC) 26–7
*Montgomery v. Lanarkshire
Health Board* 151–2
multipara
interview with Mari
Greenfield 79–80
interview with Orla Gal-
lagher 88–105

National Child Measure-
ment Programme 199
National Institute for Health and
Care Excellence (NICE) 136, 163
NHS Constitution for England 152–3
NHS Highland 30–1

Pickett, Emma 177, 178–9
plus size 11–12

Quetelet, Adolphe 16

racism
and babywear 183–4
experience of Fiona Houston 34–48
and fatphobia 55
and maternal deaths 212
rights in maternity/perinatal
services 106–9

Salmon, Nicola
interview with 51–65, 214
slings 115, 175, 181–3, 184, 185–8
String Sabina 55

Ternovszky v. Hungary 150
This Is Going to Hurt (Kay) 108
Tomiyama, Janet 27

Virgo, Vanisha
interview with 179–93, 215

water births 80–1, 118–19, 145–9
weight stigma *see also* fatphobia
in healthcare 26–9, 57, 61–2, 200–5
in maternity/perinatal services
29–33, 34–48, 55, 68–78
Wickham, Sara 135, 155, 161
World Health Organization
(WHO) 57–8, 211–12

Yeboah, Stephanie 19